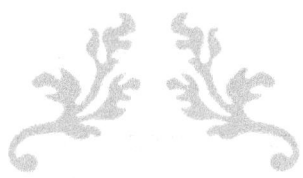

A NEW START

Your Guide to Healthful Living

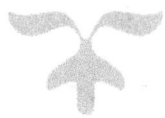

ISBN-13: 978-1500610623

ISBN-10: 1500610623
Published July, 2014

A Note from the Compiler and Distributor

This book is a compilation of information taken from various health booklets and has been used with permission.

For more information and to contact the original sources, please write to:

Character Building Books
P.O. Box 35946
London
N17 7WG

characterbuildingbooks@yahoo.co.uk

To learn more about the Distributor of this book and their ministry, please contact:

The Way Makers
Tel: 473-458-4795 (Grenada)
Tel: 917-834-6511 (USA)
Email: thewaymakers777@gmail.com

Table of Contents

Make a NEW START:
The 8 Laws of Health

Our bodies are marvellously designed and very robust, but will fail under constant exposure to abuse. The majority of the diseases we suffer today are brought about by the unhealthy lifestyle choices, which in turn form habits, then go on to form our characters. Our characters are, all said and done, what we are. Generally these choices and habits are brought on by feeling one has to submit to the peers of the day and following accepted practices of society, often without understanding their hurtful consequences.

This section of the book brings some simple rules that bring better health and happier living when applied in your life and in many cases, because of the willingness of nature, will undo much of the damage already done.

Nutrition

When a car is made, the company who makes the car writes a service manual to go with it. This informs which are the best fuel and oils for the working machinery in that car, to keep it running in the best possible condition.

In the same way, we are like machines that need good fuel to run well. Certain foods will make the best kind of blood, muscle and bone in our bodies. To keep us running well, we need to choose our foods wisely and keep our diet well balanced with the four main food groups:

1. **Fruits**
2. **Grains**
3. **Nuts and Seeds**
4. **Vegetables**

It is health to start every day in the morning with a good hearty breakfast, which could include:

- Whole Grains – like oats, whole wheat bread, brown rice or porridge
- Milks – coconut, almond or soy
- Fruits – Apples, pears, bananas, paw-paw, oranges, etc.

At midday, a good vegetable meal with:

- Starches – like potatoes, whole wheat bread and whole grains
- Protein – which is in beans, nuts and seeds
- Greens – cabbage, silverbeet, spinach, parsley, etc.
- Colors – carrots, pumpkin, cauliflower, beetroot, etc.

For the evening meal, a light fruit meal with a little grain, like cracker biscuits. The light evening meal should be eaten at least 2-3 hours before going to bed. It is also important to eat meals at regular times and not to eat between meals at all, as our stomachs need to rest as well. It is well recommended to have some raw salads with each meal also, as this aids digestion.

It is possible to have too much of a good thing. We need to have an understanding of the word "Nutrition". It means to eat foods only that are good for the up-building of our bodies and eat them in moderation, at the right times.

Fatty foods tend to store as fat which increases the risk of disease and makes us more sluggish.

Eating a good hearty breakfast, a good-sized mid-day meal and a light tea, gives us the fuel we need at the right times when we need the energy. It also helps us keep our bodies in good shape and helps in weight control.

If a good-sized meal cannot be eaten at midday, it would be wise to have more in the morning, rather than have a large heavy meal late in the day. This can result in disturbed sleep, not waking refreshed in the morning and an unhealthy circle can soon develop.

Some foods are not good for our well-being. Alcohol, smoking, coffee and drugs are very harmful. Lollies, canned drinks, ice creams, and cakes made with a high sugar content are also dangerous for our ongoing health.

Harmful effects may not be noticed straight away, but over a period of time, our immune system will began to fail. This will increase the risk of disease and may result in aged damaged organs and even death.

Eating too many sweets and sugar foods makes unhealthy blood and they are not good for building strong healthy tissues and bones, etc.

By not eating between meals, it reduces the temptation of eating sweets.

Exercise

If someone has broken an arm or leg, it needs to be put into a plaster cast for 6-8 weeks so that the bones can knit back together and heal properly.

When the plaster is removed, it can be easily noticed that the limb that was broken is smaller, paler, weaker and stiffer than the other limbs that had frequent use.

The joints of the broken limb will not move as freely as the good limb and it could be more painful to move for a time. **ONLY EXERCISE WILL BRING IT BACK TO GOOD USE AGAIN.**

This is just a picture of what happens to the whole body when we fail to get proper exercise. Each part suffers and in turn the whole body suffers.

Some people work at sedentary occupations. Even though they are brain tired at the end of the day from standing or sitting for hours in heavy concentration, they need to exercise physically and breathe fresh air deeply. It would be well for these people to enjoy some late afternoon or early morning sunshine and exercise in the garden, cycling or brisk walking.

When oxygen is lacking in the body, the blood moves sluggishly and the waste, poisonous matter that should be eliminated, is held in the body and the blood becomes impure. Exercise improves the blood circulation and helps cleanse the blood. Good health depends on good circulation.

Proper exercise gives life to the whole body. It gives strength to the digestive organs, the liver, the kidneys, the lungs and the heart. Exercise is excellent recreation not only for the body but also for the mind. It brings relief to the weary brain, helping us to think more clearly and to feel more cheerful. The whole body becomes more resistant to disease.

It is not wise to exercise too vigorously, especially after eating a larger meal. The blood is then needed in the stomach to break down the food and is not as available for the other strenuous exercise. Exercise, like all other daily activities must be done with care, thoughtfulness and common sense. Let us begin to take some steps and make a decision to get some exercise today and every day from here on.

Listed below are some benefits of good exercise:
- Prevention of heart disease
- Lowers blood pressure
- Prevention of and treatment of obesity
- Increases circulation and oxygen intake
- Improved sleep
- Increases self-worth
- Lowers cholesterol levels in the blood
- Decrease in anxiety and relief of depression
- Elevation in mood and vigour
- Stronger heart beat and lowering resting heart rate
- Increase fitness level
- Aids in stress control

Water

Water is very important to this world. About three quarters of the earth is made up of water.

Most of it is salt water but the sun has the ability to change salt water into fresh water.

Just to basically explain it – the heat from the sun picks up small drops of water from the sea and takes them up to make clouds but it leaves the salt behind.

As the clouds gather more and more moisture, the drops get heavier and heavier until they become heavier than air and fall as rain on the earth.

Also springs of fresh water bubble up from under the earth.

Often big rivers start from snow and springs in the mountains. As they trickle down to the lower areas, water from the rain and thawing snow join the streams and together they tumble downward. As different creeks join the flow, they become rivers and soon the rivers flow into the mighty ocean – to repeat the ongoing, never-ending cycle.

Water is the very important part of our lives, both inside and outside the body.

We need to drink 8-10 good-sized glasses of clean water each day. A good health habit to develop, is to drink 2-3 glasses of warm water when you get out of bed. This helps to flush out the stomach and digestion track.

It is best not to drink after 20 minutes before eating food. This way the water does not dilute the acid juices which break down the food when it comes into the stomach at meal time. For this reason it is best not to drink with any meal. It can cause the food to stay in the stomach longer than needed and it starts to ferment and build up bad gasses.

The blood needs a good supply of clean water as well. Water helps blood to flow around our blood system, to keep our body running well.

If we could follow our blood into all the hidden recesses of our body, we would find that it picks up poisons and waste matter on its travels. Water is essential for the function of the kidneys as they continuously filter the blood.

The kidneys' work is made more efficient if we drink plenty of clean water. The body will keep healthier. Also, if we have trouble with passing solid wastes (constipation), this can often be relieved by drinking a good supply of warm water.

It is essential to drink plenty of water when we are sick. It helps to pave the way for a quicker recover. People suffering from colds, fever, infections and viruses will be greatly helped if they increase their water intake.

On the outside, we must not forget that our skin is another very important organ that eliminates body wastes. A bath or shower every day cleans the skin of germs and impurities, helping all the organs to aid the body do their work.

All our clothes and bedding should be washed in clean water to keep them fresh and clean as well.

Water on the outside and the inside assists nature to keep out disease.

Sunshine

Did you ever stop to think what it would be like without sunshine on this earth? There would be no life at all, not a leaf could grow or a flower bloom. No animal could live and no fish could survive in the oceans.

It is from the mighty power and energy of the sun that all vegetable and animal life gets the power to live and grow. Some get it from the sin directly and some indirectly.

Not only does the sun give off light and heat, but its rays also kill off many germs. The sun gives plants the power to take carbon dioxide and oxygen from the air, a process called photosynthesis, and combine these into basic foods which are eaten by other living animals. This is called chlorophyll, the green substance in the leaves of the plants. This is a wonderful process that man, with all his big laboratories and expensive equipment has never been able to do, or even fully understand.

Energy from the sun's rays also acts on our skin, giving Vitamin D, one of the vitamins needed in our body.

When we wake up in the morning and the sun shines in our bedrooms, we immediately have a more cheerful "spring in our step" and a healthier glow to our faces.

The sun gives off great amounts of life healing energy each hour of every day.

Sunlight, either from shining on us directly, or from eating foods grown in the sun, assists in keeping the blood clean and pure which supplies life to each part of our body. It also strengthens the body's immune system.

Even sick people are greatly helped by relaxing in moderate amounts of sunshine and fresh air.

The sun has many healing properties that greatly benefit the health of the body:

- Aids in relieving acutely swollen arthritic joints
- Relieves certain symptoms of PMS
- Increases calcium absorption
- Forms Vitamin D
- Destroys bacteria and viruses
- Lowers blood pressure
- Brings a sense of well being
- Promotes healing of some skin irritations

Of course there is danger of over exposure to the harshness of the sun's rays, but as in all facets of our lives, it is always possible to overdo even the good.

Regulate the exposure to the sun with moderation and common sense.

Temperance

What is temperance? The simple meaning is that we need to be sensible and careful in all facets of life. Temperance covers areas of diet, sleeping habits, choice and fitting of our clothing, our daily activities, our exercise and all other aspects of our life.

Firstly in food – it is important that each day we eat a well-balanced diet. This means eating the right amounts of food from the different groups at the right times of the day. We should never feel bloated and over-full after a meal. We should always feel we could eat a little more when we leave the meal table. Due to body make-up and workload, the needs differ for each person, but the body knows and will give signals of satisfaction before getting overfull. The body does not handle food nearly as well when it is gulped down as it does when it is chewed well. It takes a little time for the stomach to give the full signal and one can easily overeat developing into a bad habit, overweight, gas and other problems. Chew the food well, let the saliva work on the contents. Remember our stomachs do not have teeth – digestion starts in the mouth.

It is unwise to mix vegetables with fruits at any one meal. Lemons and oranges will not have so bad an effect being acid fruits, but sweet fruits such as bananas, dates, raisins, etc. are a bad combination with vegetables. Temperance covers the old adage, "You can have too much of a good thing". If we continually overeat, the body becomes continually overloaded, the stomach becomes weary and the risk of disease increases.

Some illnesses will not necessarily surface immediately, but they can accumulate internally and break out once internal damage is irreversible.

Temperance in drinking is also important. Teas, coffee, canned drinks and alcohol should be out of the diet. Most certain caffeine and although it may give energy for a short term, after the boost has had its peak, the body becomes tired and the mind can become depressed. Often the low that comes after the caffeine wears off is worse than the tiredness before taking the cup of coffee. If you are tired, the body is calling for sleep, not a charge of high-octane fuel. The human machinery can only last so long and starts breaking down after continual abuse.

Clean fresh water taken up to 20-30 minutes before a meal and two hours after a meal, adding up to 8-10 glasses a day is the best beverage we can possibly have.

Clothing should fit our bodies well. It should not be tight around any part of the body to restrict blood flow or digestion functions. However, all parts of our body, including our arms, legs and head, should be well covered in colder climates, to keep the whole body warm, close fitting for safety, but not too tight. It is important to be covered neatly as well as modestly. What we wear on the outside often gives a pretty good indication of what we are like on the inside.

Sleeping is also included in temperance. One hour before midnight is better than two hours after midnight. Developing a habit of going to bed about 8:30-9:30 p.m. and rising about 5:00-6:00 a.m. will help bring health to body and mind.

Air

Did you ever stop to think that we live at the bottom of an ocean of air that surrounds the earth?

We could live a few weeks without food and a few days without water, but how long do you think we would live if we had no air?

In 1 or 2 minutes we would all become unconscious and within 5 or 6 minutes we would all be dead. We need a constant supply of pure air into our bodies to keep our blood pure and healthy, to soothe our nervous system and fill our lungs and keep our voices speaking clearly.

The first thing a baby needs when it is first born is to breathe air. Air is "life" to a new born baby and that air is essential to that little one right through life.

Children should run and play in the fresh air every day if possible. This will help them to be more cheerful, healthier, and happier.

Pure, fresh air gives a good appetite, helps improve the blood flow, purifies the blood, refreshes the body, helps digestion of food, helps us sleep soundly and also helps to heal the sick.

Our homes should be kept clean as well as being well ventilated with fresh air. Curtains and drapes should be open to allow sunshine and air to fill the rooms with life giving elements. We should also sleep with windows open at night where possible. The fresh air will help our sleep be more relaxed and restful.

If there are sick in the home, the room should not be shut up for them to breathe the same air over and over again. The oxygen in the fresh air will help bring a quicker recovery, helping the blood to cleanse and purify, resulting in greater strength and health – sooner.

Air that Refreshes

There is a kind of air that can energise and relax the mind and body within minutes. It is found near waterfalls, in forests at the beach and after a rain storm. However, there is another kind of air that can bring on anxiety, depression and even suicidal feelings.

What Makes the Difference?

Air contains positively and negatively charged molecules called ions. These ions become electrically charged as a result of gaining or losing an electron. Air containing an abundance of negative ions is refreshing, as found in the bush, or by river, lakes, waterfalls and at the beach. On the other hand, air containing mostly positive ions as found in city centres, airports, poorly ventilated rooms, and on crowded motorways, is associated with headaches, anxiety, insomnia and depression.

The blend of exercise and fresh air are important, as good active exercise increases the demand for fresh air and we naturally breathe more deeply.

Take time out of the busy day to take a walk in the bush or some other quiet place and do some deep breathing. It will not only life your chest, but life your day.

Rest

In the hustle and bustle of our busy modern lives, most of us keep going until we finally drop at the end of the day from exhaustion. We have heard of the saying "burning the candle at both ends" to describe a person who is always going full speed, borrowing from the store of energy and robbing themselves of needed rest to let body and mind rest up and refresh.

This is not the best way for us to live. Being moderate, even in creative and productive work, is what is best for our health.

The first place we think of when we speak of rest is in our beds for the evening sleep. We should get into a regular pattern. Going to bed at 8:30-9:30 p.m. is a good time for settling down to sleep and 5:00-6:00 a.m. is good for rising. This pattern brings a good night's rest and unloads pressure in the morning to beat the clock when work starts.

Quiet reading, some exercise and family time at the breakfast table brings a sweet start to the day. This may be the ideal, but not always practical for certain lifestyles, but if one is able, the pattern soon starts getting easier and life is enjoyed more fully.

It may be hard to sleep the first few evenings at the earlier time, but upon rising at the earlier time of 6:00 a.m. approximately, one will soon be looking for sleep by 8:30-9:30 p.m.

Other places of rest, rather than sleep, is out in the beauty and quietness of nature. If possible, it is good to leave the busy cities behind and seek that rest in the quietness of a country setting, beside a river, or lake, in a grove of trees, or in the mountains. Other ways can be in a good book, giving good counsel and guidance, talking to a friend, quietly taking a walk, taking time to be with the family.

When planning time out for a holiday, use time wisely and make sure the return home brings a more refreshed and "revitalised you" than before leaving.

Worry also pulls a person down and is not good for our health. It can cause insomnia, tension, loss of confidence, depression and sluggishness. Another great enemy is guilt. Guilt is likened to the mind as pain is to the body. A guilty conscience makes a restless bed fellow.

Proper rest habits contribute to our quality of life. It also adds to the length of life. Rest also improves mental and physical efficiency. During rest your body is replenished, waste products are removed and your body systems are re-energised. You are preparing for renewed activity for the day to come.

Remember – **EARLY TO BED, EARLY TO RISE, MAKE A PERSON HEALTHY AND WISE.**

Trust in Divine Power

The key to the basic eight natural doctors of health is a well-balanced, common sense outlook on life.

We need to have a complete health programme and although we can make choices to follow the healthy lifestyle, we still have weaknesses and if only we had something or someone to lean on to give strength through our problems and give us the power to overcome the fall downs. Certainly we do have friends that we can talk to for encouragement, but we need to remember that every one of us are in this together and all are struggling with our weak areas.

There is One with power that we can lean on, One who is interested in our health. Many a person from ages past, has found a NEW START, physically, mentally and spiritually when they have sought divine aid. That power comes from the compassionate Creator of the Universe, the One whose interest is in every individual's personal health. The well proven pages of the Scriptures, that has stood the test of time, bring out good healthy principles. "Beloved, I wish above all things that thou mayest prosper and be in health, even as thy soul prospereth." 3 John 2

Now, one may reason that this old stuff is for centuries past and turn away, but we need to stop and think awhile.

Doctors and modern science are finding in research that good health is more than just physical and mental, but adding the dimension of spiritual health as well. The facts ad figures that are coming from research now are amazing, they are lining up exactly with the Scripture principles. If we will keep to the eight doctors laid out in this booklet, we will have more vibrant health.

A good diet allows us to think more clearly. A clear mind helps us to make good choices and to have clear spiritual, pure thoughts. Good pure minds keep the body in trim, completing the circle of wanting good Nutrition, Exercise, Water, Temperance, Air, Rest, and will increase our Trust in Divine Power.

Yes – try a NEW START today – and everyday will start off with a NEW START and as the pattern develops, old ways will quickly drop off as the mind and body enjoy increased good health.

"Come unto me, all ye that labour and are heavy laden, and I will give you rest." – Matthew 11:28

The Place of Herbs in Rational Therapy

Originally Compiled by Elder D.E. Robinson
Secretary to Mrs. E.G. White
At "Elmshaven" Office, St. Helena, California
May 26, 1931, Revised October 18, 1934

INTRODUCTION

In June, 1863, at Otsego, Michigan, Mrs. E.G. White was given a vision, in which she received much previous instruction for the church regarding the preservation of health and principles of rational treatment of disease. During subsequent years, she wrote and published hundreds of pages on this subject.

In articles for the papers, in a number of books, and in manuscripts and letters, Mrs. White set forth principles of healthful living that have stood the test of time and scientific research. She pointed out the evils of the common use of poisonous drugs in medical practice, and urged the value of nature's remedies, sunlight, fresh air, healthful food, pure water, exercise, rest, and the value of water as a means of applying heat and cold in the treatment of disease.

The few statements regarding herbs that are found in Mrs. White's writings, are clear and definite. She says that "there are simple herbs that can be used for the recovery of the sick;" that there are certain "herbs that are harmless, the use of which will tide over many apparently serious difficulties;" and that "leave no injurious effects in the system" as do drugs.

It is not a fact that God has been calling His people to a system of therapy in which, contrary to general ideas and custom, the administration of any kind of medicinal doses, should play only a minor part. First emphasis is given to ascertaining and removing the cause of sickness, and the methods of treatment that are urged in the Testimonies are such as will give nature an opportunity to carry forward the healing processes.

It should also be noted that in recommending herbs as a therapeutic agency in disease, Mrs. White placed the emphasis upon their intelligent use in the home rather than upon their being prescribed by physicians. This, however, does not remove from the conscientious physician his responsibility to learn what he can regarding the benefits of such simple herbs.

In the following quotations, the statements relative to the use of herbs are indicated by italics, but appear in their full setting, that the reader may note the arraignment of the drugging system connected and contrasted with the recommended use of herbs.

Elder D.E. Robinson

The Place of Herbs in Rational Therapy

Statements Written by Mrs. E.G. White (Italics ours, Editor)

PRAYER, FAITH AND REMEDIES

(1) "In regard to the matter of prayer for the sick, many confusing ideas are advanced. One says, He who has been prayed for must walk out in faith, giving God the glory, and making use of no remedies. If he is at a health institute, he should leave it at once. I know that these ideas are wrong, and that if accepted, they would lead to many evils. {PH144 4.1}

"On the other hand, I do not wish to say anything that might be interpreted to mean a lack of belief in the efficacy of prayer. The path of faith lies close beside the path of presumption. {PH144 4.2}

"It is no denial of faith to use rational remedies judiciously. Water, air, and sunshine, these are God's healing agencies. {PH144 4.3}

"The use of certain herbs that the Lord has made to grow for the good of man, is in harmony with the exercise of faith,"—Manuscript 31, 1911 (written June 3, 1888). {PH144 4.4}

Learn To (Do for Yourself)

(2) "Now in regard to that which we can do for ourselves: There is a point that requires careful, thoughtful consideration. I must become acquainted with myself. I must be a learner always as to how to take care of this building, the body God has given me, that I may preserve it in the very best condition of health. I must eat those things which will be for my very best good physically and I must take special care to have my clothing such as will conduce to a healthful circulation of the blood. I must not deprive myself of exercise and air. I must get all the sunlight that it is possible for me to obtain. {PH144 5.1}

"I must have wisdom to be a faithful guardian of my body. I should do a very unwise thing to enter a cool room when in a perspiration; I should show myself an unwise steward to allow myself to sit in a draught, and thus expose myself so as to take cold. I should be unwise to sit with cold feet and limbs and thus drive back the blood from the extremities to the brain or internal organs. I should always protect my feet in damp weather. {PH144 5.2}

"I should eat regularly of the most healthful food which will make the best quality of blood, and I should not work intemperately if it is in my power to avoid doing so. {PH144 5.3}

"And when I violate the laws God has established in my being, I am to repent and reform, and place myself in the most favorable condition under the doctors God has provided,—pure air, pure water, and the healing, precious sunlight. Water can be used in many ways to relieve suffering. Draughts of clear, hot water taken before eating (half a quart more or less), will never do any harm, but will rather be productive of good. *A cup of tea made from catnip herb will quiet the nerves.* {PH144 6.1}

USEFUL REMEDIES

"Hop tea will induce sleep. Hop poultices over the stomach will relieve pain. {PH144 6.2}

"If the eyes are weak, if there is pain in the eyes, or inflammation, soft flannel cloths wet in hot water and salt, will bring relief quickly. {PH144 6.3}

"When the head is congested, if the feet and limbs are put in a bath with a little mustard, relief will be obtained. {PH144 6.4}

"There are many more simple remedies, which will do much to restore healthful action to the body. All these simple preparations the Lord expects us to use for ourselves; but man's extremities are God's opportunities. {PH144 6.5}

"If we neglect to do that which is within the reach of nearly ever family, and ask the Lord to relieve pain, when we are too indolent to make use of these remedies within our power, it is simply presumption. The Lord expects us to work in order that we may obtain food. He does not propose that we shall gather the harvest unless we break the sod, till the soil, and cultivate the produce. Then God sends the rain and the sunshine and the clouds to cause vegetation to flourish. God works, and man cooperates with God. Then there is seed time and harvest. {PH144 7.1}

"God has caused to grow out of the ground herbs for the use of man and if we understand the nature of these roots and herbs, and make a right use of them, there would not be a necessity of running for the doctor so frequently, and people would be in much better health than they are today. {PH144 7.2}

"I believe in calling upon the Great Physician when we have used the remedies I have mentioned. In regard to manner of labor we certainly need to be wise as serpents and harmless as doves. We might be very zealous, but it might be an unwise zeal, and serve to hedge up our way. Then there is danger of being so circumscribed in our work as to do very little good."—Letter 35, February 6, 1890. {PH144 7.3}

(3) "The simpler remedies are less harmful (than drug poisons) in proportion to their simplicity, but in very many cases these are used when not at all necessary. {PH144 8.1}

EVERY FAMILY TO USE HERBS

"There are simple herbs and roots that every family may use for themselves, and need not call in a physician any sooner than they would call a lawyer. {PH144 8.2}

"I do not think that I can give you any definite line of medicines compounded and dealt out by doctors that are perfectly harmless. And yet it would not be wisdom to engage in controversy over this subject. The practitioners are very much in earnest in using their dangerous concoctions; and I am decidedly opposed to resorting to such things. They never cure; they may change the difficulty to create a worse one. Many of those who practice the prescribing of drugs, would not take the same, or give them to their children. If they have an intelligent knowledge of the human body ... they must know that we are fearfully and wonderfully made, and that not a particle of these strong drugs should be introduced into this human living organism. {PH144 8.3}

"As the matter was laid open before me,,and the sad burden of the result of drug medication, the light was given me that Seventh-day Adventists should establish health institutions, discarding all these health-destroying inventions, and physicians should treat the sick upon hygienic principles."—Letter 17a, 1893 (written October 2, 1893) {PH144 8.4}

(4) "The intricate names given the medicines are used to cover up the matter, so that none will know what is given them as remedies unless they obtain a dictionary to find out the meaning of these names. {PH144 9.1}

"The Lord has given some simple herbs of the field that at times are beneficial; and if every family were educated in how to use these herbs in case of sickness, much suffering might be prevented, and no doctor need be called. These old-fashioned, simple herbs, used intelligently, would have recovered many sick, who have died under drug medication."—Letter 82, 1897 (written February 10, 1897)

HERBS HARMLESS, DRUGS HARMFUL {PH144 9}

(5) "Were I sick, I would just as soon call in a lawyer as a physician from among general practitioners. I would not touch their nostrums to which they give Latin names. I am determined to know, in straight English, the name of everything that I introduce into my system. {PH144 9.3}

"Those who make a practice of taking drugs, sin against their intelligence and endanger their whole after life. {PH144 10.1}

"There are herbs that are harmless, the use of which will tide over many apparently serious difficulties. {PH144 10.2}

"But if all would seek to become intelligent in regard to their bodily necessities, sickness would be rare instead of common. An ounce of prevention is worth a pound of cure."—Manuscript 86, 1897. (written August 25, 1897) {PH144 10.3}

(6) "Drug medication is to be discarded. On this point the conscience of the physician must ever be kept tender, and true, and clean. The inclination to use poisonous drugs, which kill, if they do not cure, needs to be guarded against. Matters have been laid open before me in reference to the use of drugs. Many have been treated with drugs, and the result has been death. Our physicians, by practicing drug medication, have lost many cases that need not have died if they had left their drugs out of the sick-room. {PH144 10.4}

DRUGS KILL

"Fever cases have been lost, when had the physicians left off entirely their drug treatment, had they put their wits to work, and wisely and persistently used the Lord's own remedies, plenty of air and water, the patients would have recovered. The reckless use of these things that should be discarded has decided the case of the sick. {PH144 10.5}

"Experimenting in drugs is a very expensive business. Paralysis of the brain and tongue is often the result, and the victims die an unnatural death, when, if they had been treated perseveringly with unwearied, unrelaxed diligence, with hot and cold water, hot compresses, packs and dripping sheets, they would be alive today. {PH144 11.1}

Learn God's Methods

"Nothing should be put into the human system that will leave a baleful influence behind. And to carry out the light on this subject, to practice hygienic treatment, is the reason which has been given me for establishing sanitariums in various localities.... {PH144 11.2}

"We must become enlightened on these subjects. The intricate names given medicine are used to cover up the matter, so that none will know what is given them as remedies unless they consult a dictionary. {PH144 11.3}

(7) "As to drugs being used in our institutions, it is contrary to the light which the Lord has been pleased to give. The drugging business has done more harm to our world and killed more than it has helped or cured. The light was first given to me why institutions should be established, that is sanitariums were to reform the medical practices of physicians. {PH144 12.1}

"This is God's method. The herbs that grow for the benefit of man, and the little handful of herbs kept and steeped and used for sudden ailments, have served tenfold, yes, one hundred fold better purposes, than all the drugs hidden under mysterious names and dealt out to the sick. {PH144 12.2}

"It is a delusion and a farce, and the Lord has revealed to me that this practice would not preserve life, but would introduce into the system those things which should never be there, for they would do a deleterious work on the human organism."—Letter 59, 1898 (written August 29, 1898) {PH144 12.3}

(8) "The drug science has been exalted, but if every bottle that comes from every such institution were done away with, there would be fewer invalids in the world today. Drug medication should never have been introduced into our institutions. There was no need of this being so, and for this very reason the Lord would have us establish an institution where He can come in and where His grace and power can be revealed. 'I am the Resurrection and the Life,' He declares. {PH144 12.4}

LEARN TO TREAT YOURSELF

"The true method for healing the sick is to tell them of the herbs that grow for the benefit of man. Scientists have attached large names to these simplest preparations, but true education will lead us to teach the sick that they need not call in a doctor any more than they would call in a lawyer. They can themselves administer the simple herbs if necessary. {PH144 13.1}

"To educate the human family that the doctor alone knows all the ills of infants and persons of every age is false teaching, and the sooner we as a people stand on the principles of health reform, the greater will be the blessing that will come to those who would do true medical work. There is a work to be done in treating the sick with water and teaching them to make the most of the sunshine and physical exercise. Thus in simple language, we may teach the people how to preserve health, how to avoid sickness. This is the work our sanitariums are called upon to do. This is true science."—Manuscript 105, 1898, (written August 26, 1898) {PH144 13.2}

DISCARD HUMAN CONCOCTIONS

(9) "Shall physicians continue to resort to drugs, which leave a deadly evil in the system, destroying that life which Christ came to restore? Christ's remedies cleanse the system. But Satan has tempted man to introduce into the system that which weakens the human machinery, clogging and destroying the fine, beautiful arrangements of God. The drugs administered to the sick do not restore, but destroy. Drugs never cure. Instead, they place in the system seeds which bear a very bitter harvest. {PH144 14.1}

"Our Saviour is the restorer of the moral image of God in man. He has supplied in the natural world remedies for the ills of man, that His followers may have life, and that they may have it more abundantly. We can with safety discard the concoctions which man has used in the past. The Lord has provided antidotes for disease in simple plants, and these can be used by faith, with no denial of faith; for by using the blessings provided by God for our benefit we are cooperating with Him. We can use water and sunshine and the herbs which He has caused to grow for healing maladies brought on by indiscretion or accident."—Manuscript 65, 1899. (written April 25, 1899) {PH144 14.2}

(10) "It would have been better if from the first all drugs had been kept out of our sanitariums, and use had been made of such simple remedies as are found in pure water, pure air, sunlight, and some of the simple herbs growing in the field. These would be just as efficacious as the drugs used under mysterious names, and concocted by human science, and they would leave no injurious effects in the system. {PH144 15.1}

"Thousands who are afflicted might recover their health if, instead of depending upon the drug store for their life, they would discard all drugs, and live simply, without using tea, coffee, liquor, or spices, which irritate the stomach, and leave it weak, unable to digest even simple food without stimulation."—Manuscript 115, 1903 (written September 4, 1902). {PH144 15.2}

(11) "We have been instructed that in our treatment of the sick we should discard the use of drugs. {PH144 15.3}

"There are simple herbs that can be used for the recovery of the sick, whose effect upon the system is very different from that of those drugs that poison the blood and endanger life."—Manuscript 73, 1908. {PH144 15.4}

(12) "I have been shown that we should have many more women who can deal especially with the diseases of women, many more lady nurses who will treat the sick in a simple way and without the use of drugs. {PH144 16.1}

NURSES LEARN TO USE HERBS

"There are many simple herbs which, if our nurses would learn the value of, they could use in the place of drugs, and find very effective."—Letter 90, 1908. {PH144 16.2}

"By His own working agencies He has created material which will restore the sick to health. If men would use aright the wisdom God has given them, this world would be a place resembling heaven."—Manuscript 63, 1899. {PH144 16.3}

"We should make decided efforts to heed the directions the Lord has given in regard to the care of the sick. They should be given every advantage possible. All the restorative agencies that the Lord has provided should be made use of in our sanitarium work."—Manuscript 19, 1911. {PH144 16.4}

FIGS USED ON MALIGNANT SORE

"When the Lord told Hezekiah that He would spare his life for fifteen years, and as a sign that He would fulfill His promise, caused,the sun to go back ten degrees, why did He not put His direct, restoring power upon the King? He told him to apply a bunch of figs to his sore, and that natural remedy, blessed by God, healed him. The God of nature directs the human agent to use natural remedies now."—Letter 182, 1899. {PH144 16.5}

CONTINUE HEALTH REFORM

"Special instruction should be given in the art of treating the sick, without the use of poisonous drugs, and in harmony with the light that God has given. Students should come forth from the school without having sacrificed the principles of health reform."—Letter 90, 1908. {PH144 17.1}

PHYSICIANS TO TEACH LAITY

"Those who desire to become missionaries are to hear instruction from competent physicians, who will teach them how to care for the sick, without the use of drugs. Such lessons will be of the highest value to those who go out to labor in foreign countries. And the simple remedies used will save many lives."—Manuscript 83, 1908. {PH144 17.2}

"The Lord will be the Helper of every physician who will work together with Him,in the effort to restore suffering humanity to health, not with drugs, but with nature's remedies. Christ is the great physician, the wonderful Healer. He gives success to those who work in partnership with Him."—Letter 142, 1902. {PH144 17.3}

"While the physician uses nature's remedies for physical disease, he should point his patients to Him who can relieve the maladies of both the soul and the body."—The Ministry of Healing, 111. {PH144 18.1}

"In case of sickness, the cause should be ascertained, unhealthful conditions should be changed, wrong habits corrected. Then nature is to be assisted in her effort to expel impurities and to re-establish right conditions in the system."—The Ministry of Healing, 127 {PH144 18.2}

OTHER SIMPLE REMEDIES

"Pure air, sunlight, abstemiousness, rest, exercise, proper diet, the use of water, trust in divine power,—these are the true remedies."—The Ministry of Healing, 127. {PH144 18.3}

"There are many ways of practising the healing art; but there is only one way that Heaven approves. God's remedies are the simple agencies of nature, that will not tax or, debilitate the system through their powerful properties. Pure air and water, cleanliness, a proper diet, purity of life, and a firm trust in God, are remedies for the want of which thousands are dying.... Fresh air, exercise, pure water, and clean sweet premises, are within the reach of all."— Testimonies for the Church 5:443. {PH144 18.4}

"The physician needs more than human wisdom and power that he may know how to minister to the many perplexing cases of disease of the mind and heart with which he is called to deal. If he is ignorant of the power of divine grace, he cannot help the afflicted one, but will aggravate the difficulty; but if he has a firm hold upon God, he will be able to help the diseased, distracted mind."— Testimonies for the Church 5:444. {PH144 19.1}

RATIONAL TREATMENT FOR PNEUMONIA

(13) "In the winter of 1864, my Willie was suddenly and violently brought down with lung fever. We had just buried our oldest son with this disease, and were very anxious in regard to Willie, fearing

that he, too, might die. We decided that we would not send for a physician, but do the best we could with him ourselves by the use of water, and entreat the Lord in behalf of the child. We called in a few, who had faith to unite their prayers with ours. We had a sweet assurance of God's presence and blessing. {PH144 19.2}

"The next day Willie was very sick. He was wandering. He did not seem to see or hear me when I spoke to him. His heart had no regular beat, but was in a constant agitated flutter. We continued to look to God in his behalf, and to use water freely upon his head, and a compress constantly upon his lungs, and soon he seemed as rational as ever. He suffered severe pain in his right side, and could not lie upon it for a moment. This pain we subdued with cold water compresses, varying the temperature of the water according to the degree of the fever. We were very careful to keep his hands and feet warm. {PH144 20.1}

"We expected the crisis would come the seventh day. We had but little rest during his sickness, and were obliged to give him up into other's care the fourth and fifth nights. My husband and myself the fifth day felt very anxious. The child raised fresh blood and coughed considerably. My husband spent much time in prayer. We left our child in careful hands that night. Before retiring my husband prayed long and earnestly. Suddenly his burden of prayer left him, and it seemed as though a voice spoke to him, and said,,Go lie down, I will take care of the child. {PH144 20.2}

"I had retired sick, and could not sleep for anxiety for several hours. I felt pressed for breath, Although sleeping in a large chamber, I arose and opened the door into a large hall, and was at once relieved, and soon slept. I dreamed that an experienced physician was standing by my child, watching every breath, with one hand over his heart, and with the other feeling his pulse. He turned to us and said, 'The crisis has passed. He has seen his worst night. He will now come up speedily, for he has not the injurious influence of drugs to recover from. Nature has nobly done her work to rid the system of impurities.' I related to him my worn-out condition, my pressure for breath, and the relief obtained by opening the door. {PH144 21.1}

FRESH AIR

"Said he, 'That which gave you relief will also receive your child. He needs air. You have kept him too warm. The heated air coming from a stove is injurious, and were it not for the air coming in at the crevices of the windows, would be poisonous and destroy life. (Sic.) Stove heat destroys the vitality of the air, and weakens the lungs. The child's,lungs have been weakened by the room being kept too warm. Sick persons are debilitated by disease, and need all the invigorating air that they can bear to strengthen the vital organs to resist disease. And yet in most cases, air and light are excluded from the sick room at the very time when most needed, as though dangerous enemies.' {PH144 21.2}

"This dream and my husband's experience were a consolation to us both. We found in the morning that our boy had passed a restless night. He seemed to be in a high fever until noon. Then the fever left him, and he appeared quite well, except weak. He had eaten but one small cracker through his five days sickness. He came up rapidly, and has had better health than he has had for several days before. This experience is valuable to us."—"Facts of Faith." pages 151-153. {PH144 22.1}

EXPERIENCE WITH CHARCOAL

(14) "A brother was taken sick, with inflammation of the bowels and bloody dysentery. The man was not a careful health reformer, but indulged his appetite. We were just preparing to leave Texas, where we had been laboring for several months, and we had carriages prepared to take away his brother and his family, and several others

who were suffering from malarial fever. My husband and I thought we would stand this expense rather than have the heads of several families die and leave their wives and children unprovided for. Two or three were taken in a large spring wagon on spring mattresses. {PH144 22.2}

"But this man who was suffering from inflammation of the bowels, sent for me to come to him. My husband and I decided that it would not do to move him. Fears were entertained that mortification had set in. Then the thought came to me like a communication from the Lord, to take pulverized charcoal, put water upon it, and give this water to the sick man to drink, putting bandages of the charcoal over the bowels and stomach. We were about one mile from the city of Dennison, but the sick man's son went to a blacksmith's shop, secured the charcoal, and pulverized it, and then used it according to the directions given. The result was that in half an hour there was a change for the better. We had to go on our journey and leave the family behind, but what was our surprise the following day to see their wagon overtake us. The sick man was lying in a bed in the wagon. The blessing of God had worked with the simple means used."—Letter 182, 1899. {PH144 23.1}

CHARCOAL AND SMARTWEED

"One of the most beneficial remedies is pulverized charcoal in a bag and used in fomentations. This is a most successful remedy. If wet in smartweed, boiled, it is still better. I have ordered this in cases where the sick were suffering great pain, and when it has been confided to me by the physician that he thought it was the last before the close of life. Then I suggested the charcoal, and the patient has slept, the turning point came, and recovery was the result. To students, when injured with bruised hands, and suffering with inflammation, I have prescribed this simple remedy with perfect success. The poison of inflammation is overcome, the pain removed, and healing goes on rapidly. The more severe inflammation of the eyes will be relieved by a poultice of charcoal, put in a bag and dipped in hot or cold water as will best suit the case. This works, like a charm. {PH144 24.1}

"I expect you will laugh at this; but if I could give this remedy some outlandish name that no one knew but myself, it would have greater influence."—Letter 82, 1897. {PH144 24.2}

CHARCOAL AND OLIVE OIL

"I will tell you a little about my experience with charcoal as a remedy. For some forms of indigestion, it is more efficacious than drugs. A little olive oil into which some of this powder has been stirred, tends to cleanse and heal. I find it is excellent.... {PH144 24.3}

"Always study and teach the use of the simplest remedies, and the special blessing of the Lord may be expected to follow the use of these means which are within the reach of the common people."— Letter 100, 1903. {PH144 25.1}

PINE, CEDAR, AND FIR

(15) "Light was given that there is health in the fragrance of the pine, the cedar, and the fir. And there are several other kinds of trees that have medicinal properties that are health promoting."— Letter 95, 1902 (Written June 26, 1902) {PH144 25.2}

THE USE OF CHARCOAL FOR INFLAMMATION INSECT BITES, ETC.

"On one occasion a physician came to me in great distress. He had been called to attend a young woman who was dangerously ill. She had contracted fever while on the campground and was taken to our school-building, near Melbourne, Australia. But she became so much worse that it was feared she could not live. The physician, Dr. Merritt Kellogg came to me and said, 'Sister White, have you any light for me on this case? If relief cannot be given our sister, she can live but a few hours.' I replied, 'Send to a blacksmith's shop and get some pulverized charcoal; make a poultice of it, and lay it over her stomach and sides.' The doctor hastened away to follow out my instructions. Soon he returned, saying, 'Relief came in less than half an hour after the application of the poultices. She is now having the first natural sleep she has had for days.' {PH144 25.3}

"I have ordered the same treatment for others who were suffering great pain, and it has brought relief, and been the means of saving life. My mother had told me that snake bites and the sting of reptiles and poisonous insects could often be rendered harmless by the use of charcoal poultices. When working on the land at Avondale, Australia, the workmen would often bruise their hands and limbs, and this in many cases resulted in such severe inflammation that the worker would have to leave his work for some time. One came to me one day in this condition, with his hand tied in a sling. He was much troubled over the circumstances; for his help was needed in clearing the land. I said to him, 'Go to the place where you have been burning the timber, and get me some charcoal from the eucalyptus tree, and pulverize it, and I will dress your hand.' This was done, and the next morning he reported that the pain was gone. Soon he was ready to return to his work. {PH144 26.1}

"I write these things that you may know that the Lord has not left us without the use of simple remedies which when used will not leave the system in the weakened condition in which the use of drugs so often leave it. We need well trained nurses who can understand how to use the simple remedies that nature provides for restoration to health, and who can teach those who are ignorant of the laws of health how to use these simple but effective cures."—Letter 90, 1908. {PH144 27.1}

End of Quotations from D.E. Robinson's compilation.

SUPPLEMENT

Inspired Research Sources for Medical Missionary Work

The International Nutrition Research Institute was held June 7-11 at Arlington, California. There, authentic information was given for Medical Missionary work and preparing for the time of trouble. This was especially appropriate for this time for, "soon there will be no work done in ministerial lines except medical missionary work." CH 533

Therefore we should begin now preparing for the future. What is the use of preparing for the past? At this institute, Loma Linda doctors and other research workers gave us unbiased results of their research and not mere vindicating of opinions grown venerable with age.

History of Natural Hygiene: The College History Teachers met at the same time as the nutrition group, and Dr. E.K. Vande Vere of E.M.C., Berrien Springs, Michigan, gave a study all afternoon on the Natural Hygiene movement, culminating in the work of Doctors Jennings, Graham, Trall, Jackson and others. Then Brother Arthur White gave a lectures showing the relation of their work to our denominational health program in Battle Creek and other institutions. When Mrs. E.G. White was shown her vision on the health work in 1863, she wrote it out in the book, *How to Live,* and over half of that book consisted of quotations from the Natural Hygiene doctors, for she found in their books the technical details that harmonized with the principles she had written out. They discarded drugs and used water treatments, massage, vegetarian diet and herbs. This was generally adopted in our early work, and later taken over by the Nature Cure and Herbalist and similar schools of medicine. This throws light on Dr. David Paulson's compilation of Testimonies as follows:

Drugs Not Recommended: "You are not justified in advocating one school above the others as if it were the only one worthy of respect. Those who vindicate one school of medicine and bitterly condemn another, are actuated by a zeal that is not according to knowledge. With Pharisaic pride some men look down upon others who have received a diploma from the so-called standard school.... The use of drugs has resulted in far more harm than good, and should our physicians who claim to believe the truth, almost entirely dispense with medicine, and faithfully practice along the line of *hygiene*, using *nature's remedies*, far greater success would attend their efforts. There is no need whatever to exalt the method whereby drugs are administered. I know whereof I speak. Brethren of the medical profession, I entreat you to think candidly and put away childish things.... They resort to drugs when greater skill and knowledge would teach them the *more excellent way*." Extracts on Medical Work, pages 19-23. Also Loma Linda Messages, page 62, it says:

ALL SHOULD STUDY

"The truth for this time, the third angel's message, is to be proclaimed with a loud voice as we approach the great final test. This *test must come* to the churches in connection with *true medical missionary work*." We are told that in time of trouble "there will be sick ones, plenty of them, that will need help" so because of the need, but also "for their own sake, they should, while they have opportunity, become intelligent in regard to disease, its causes, prevention and cure, and those who will do this will find a field of labor anywhere." Counsels on Health, 506.

"Let them prepare themselves for usefulness by studying the books that have been written for our instruction in these lines. Form *Reading Circles*...lay aside the busy cares of the day and unite in study.' 7T 62-67. There we have an inspired program for preparing for the time of trouble.

Weight Control
Some Genuine Help

WHAT IS OBESITY?

Being **overweight** means a person has an excess body weight compared to set standards. **Obesity** refers more specifically to an abnormally high proportion of body fat. Many people who are overweight are also obese.

The most commonly used method of measuring an ideal body weight is the body mass index (BMI). This calculation is based on height and weight and is not gender-specific. It is found by dividing a person's weight in kilograms by height in meters squared. The mathematical formula is: **weight (kg)/height squared (m^2).**

A person is considered to be in a healthy weight range for their height if their BMI is between 19 and 24. They would be considered overweight with a BMI of 25-29 and doctors define any BMI at 30 or higher to be obesity.

The World Health Organization recognises obesity is the biggest unrecognised health problem in the world. This problem has reached epidemic proportions globally, with more than 1 billion adults being overweight and at least 300 million of them clinically obese. Current obesity levels range from below 5% in China, Japan and certain African nations, to over 75% in urban Samoa. But even in relatively low prevalence countries like China, rates are almost 20% in some cities.

Of especial concern is the increasing incidence of child obesity. An estimated 17.6 million children under five are estimated to be overweight worldwide. A national children's survey in New Zealand has found that 31% of children are either overweight or obese.

The economic burden of obesity accounts for 2-6% of total health care costs in several developed countries; some estimates put the figure as high as 7%.

FACTORS CONTRIBUTING TO OBESITY

Research on both animals and humans shows that the two major contributors to obesity are physical inactivity and a high-fat diet. In the U.S., overeating and sedentary living are encouraged despite contradictory messages that promote being slim. Today, large numbers of well-advertised, affordable fast foods not only encourage overeating, but are nutritionally unbalanced and high in calories. Senator George McGovern called obesity "paradoxically enough...the number One malnutrition problem in the United States."

Most modern programs unwittingly promote overeating and appetite by keeping dieters preoccupied with food – counting calories, measuring food, and preparing tempting, low calorie dishes. By beholding, we become changed. Thus, the more one preoccupies oneself with food, the more intense will be the temptation to overeat or crave unhealthful food.

HEALTH RISKS OF OBESITY

The health risks of obesity have been officially recognised since about 1985/1986. Some who are at a "healthy weight" may still have health risks due to their body fat distribution. In the U.S., obesity is a major contributor to 5 out of the top 10 killer diseases:

- Heart disease
- Cancer
- Stroke
- Diabetes
- Atherosclerosis

Obesity is also associated with an increased risk for the following conditions:

- Hypertension
- Gallstones
- Gout
- Degenerative joint disease of the hips and knees
- Fatty liver
- Fungal and yeast infections of the skin
- Varicose veins
- Sleep apnea
- Increased levels of total cholesterol
- Triglycerides and low density lipoproteins (often referred to as "bad cholesterol")
- Decreased levels of high density lipoproteins (often referred to as "good" cholesterol)
- Reduced fertility
- Menstrual irregularities
- High risk pregnancies
- Decreased mobility
- Increased surgical risks

Careful evaluation of the Framingham data gives no indication that there is a "safe" level of overweight, that weight gain after middle age in health or that desirable weights increase with age.

The 26-year study of over 8,000 non-drinking, non-smoking Seventh Day Adventist men showed that very lean men had the lowest risk for deaths from heart disease, cancer and stroke. The average age of death was 80.5 years in the lowest weight group and 75.8 years in the highest weight group.

Keeping slim delays the age of the onset of initial menstruation (menarche). Women who mature early are more obese than women reaching puberty later. In women, fat tissue is a significant source of extra gonadal oestrogen (gonadal source of oestrogen in the ovaries).

Fat accounts for about one third of the circulating oestrogen in premenopausal women and the primary source of oestrogen in postmenopausal women. Furthermore, thin women produce a less potent form of oestrogen, while obese women produce a more potent oestrogen, while obese women produce a more potent oestrogen. Oestrogen has been linked to cancer of the breast and reproductive system. Girls who reach puberty earlier may be at greater risk for certain cancers because they may be exposed to both higher and more potent oestrogen levels for a longer time period.

As previously mentioned, the health risks of obesity are related not only to weight and total fat but also to the pattern of weight distribution. An excess of fat in the abdominal or upper body area (apple-shaped distribution) is associated with greater health risks than fat in the lower body are (pear-shaped distribution).

Studies show that upper body obesity correlated highly with heart disease, stroke diabetes and death, independent of the degree of obesity. Studies have also shown that breast and uterine cancer correlate with increased upper body fat distribution.

Although smokers weigh less than non-smokers, they have an increased (more dangerous) waist/hip ratio. Furthermore, when smokers stop smoking, the fat distribution is likely to improve in spite of some weight gain.

Weight cycling and the yo-yo syndrome are the names given to repeated loss and gain. Persons with high weight variability are 25-100 percent more likely to be victims of heart disease and premature death than those who maintain a stable weight.

Furthermore, it may be just as deleterious to lose the same 2 kg 10 times as to lose 22kg and regain it once.

Significant psychological problems associated with obesity include: anxiety, depression and poor self-image. Obsession with weight control (especially in women) has led to radical dieting and to a growing epidemic of eating disorders such as bulimia and anorexia nervosa.

In summary, overweight people need to lose weight and keep it off. Excess pounds take years off their lives by directly causing major disease by intensifying nearly all health problems, by complicating surgery and by requiring more potent medication. A body weight of at least 10 percent lower than the U.S. average is associated with lower death rates. Maintaining a healthy body weight throughout life promoted good health returns – improved quality of life, increased energy and mobility, and peace of mind.

METHODS OF WEIGHT CONTROL
Many individuals attempt to lose weight by the following methods:

- Calorie restriction
- Exercise
- Behaviour modification
- Surgery
- Drugs
- Any combination of the above methods

Dr. Theodore Van Itallie said, "The reason we have so many diet program types is that none of them really work." Participants who remain on weight loss programs typically lose approximately 10 percent of their body weight. Sadly, 90-95 percent of weight loss programs ultimately fail. A troublesome problem in obesity management is that with long-term calorie restriction, the body become more energy efficient. As a result, the more weight one loses, the more difficult it becomes to lose.

In addition to the health hazards associated with obesity, there are equally hazardous effects from very rapid weight loss programs or starvation diets. These effects include the following:

- Heart disorders
- Gallstones
- Gouty arthritis
- Fainting/weakness
- Fatigue
- Muscle cramps
- Headache
- Nausea
- Diarrhea/constipation
- Elevated cholesterol
- Uric acid levels
- Changes in liver function
- Anemia
- Edema or fluid retention
- Cold intolerance
- Dry skin
- Hair loss
- Loss of menstrual periods
- Decreased libido
- Personality changes
- Even death

Chronic dieting in itself can cause psychological harm. Chronic dieters are easily upset, emotional, subject to mood swings and are more likely to eat when anxious. They have trouble with concentration, have lost touch with hunger signals and satiety satisfaction, have low self-esteem and are eager to please others.

HARMFUL EFFECTS OF OVEREATING

Overeating, even of "healthful" food, has serious physiological consequences for both body and brain in the following ways:

- Weakens digestive organs
- Worsens pre-existing disease
- Decreases vitality of both body and brain
- Causes headaches
- Causes indigestion/colic
- Causes bad breath
- Promotes cravings for unhealthy quality and quantity of food
- Decreases mental alertness
- Promotes unclear thinking
- Has a depressing influence on the mind
- Lessens spiritual discernment

We need less of temporal food and more "spiritual" food – more of the bread of life. The simpler our diet, the better it will be for all of us. Paul felt a responsibility to preserve all his powers to the glory of God. He wrote, *"And every man that striveth for the mastery is temperate in all things...I keep under my body, and bring it into subjection lest that by any means, when I have preached to others, I myself should be cast away."* 1 Corinthians 9:25, 27

LIFESTYLE CHANGES THAT PROMOTE IDEAL BODY WEIGHT

Overweight people share the following problems:

- They think too much about food
- They eat too often
- They do not stop eating once they start
- They do not get adequate exercise

Here are some suggestions for lifestyle improvements that will help these problems and lead to ideal body weight without radical dieting or deprivation.

1. Eat a variety of unrefined, high-fibre foods from the following food groups: fruits, vegetables, whole grains, legumes, some seeds and nuts. Eat a larger portion of the low-calorie foods such as greens, tomatoes and cucumbers. Eat more moderately of such foods as: dried fruits, pumpkin, beans, potatoes and whole grain cereals.

2. Avoid rich, refined foods such as: fats (margarine, butter, mayonnaise, etc.), cooking oils, fried foods, sugar/syrup, hot spicy foods or too much salt. Learn to cook for adequate nutrition without the use of meat and dairy products. The medical literature indicated that serious food-borne illness – largely from animal products – is increasing yearly. All of the above foods listed tend to encourage cravings and overeating.

3. Eat slowly and chew well. Take time to enjoy your meal.

4. Have regular mealtime with no between-meal snacks. For best digestion, mealtimes should be at least 5 hours apart.

5. Breakfast should be the largest meal of the day. Supper, if any, should be the lightest meal of the day. Two meals per day is ideal – skipping the evening meal entirely. Fast for 24 hours one day a week (Eat breakfast then do not eat until the next breakfast time).

6. Get plenty of rest, as peaceful sleep is a potent restorer of both body and mind. Have regular bedtime hours before 10 pm. The best restorative sleep occurs in the pre-midnight hours.

7. The most effective exercise is brisk walking or gardening outdoors in the fresh air and sunlight. The ideal time for most efficient burning of calories is for 20-30 minutes within two hours after mealtime.

8. The beverage that best meets the body's physiological needs, quenches thirst, and removes many cravings is

water. The body requires approximately 2.25 litres per day in order to perform its functions well. Drink enough to keep the color of the urine pale. The best time to drink your water is between mealtimes. Drink no later than a ½ hour before eating and 1 ½ - 2 hours after mealtime. Drinking large quantities of liquids with the meal hinders digestion in the following ways:

    i.   If the liquid is cold, the stomach must first spend energy warming it up,

    ii. The liquid must be absorbed before the stomach can begin the digestive process.

9. Avoid entirely nicotine (tobacco in all forms), alcohol, caffeine and caffeine-related compounds (theobromine in chocolate and theophylline in tea). Studies have shown that both smoking and high alcohol consumption may be the major contributors to the development of upper body or abdominal fat distribution. The inhibitory nerves of the brain's frontal lobes are the most sensitive to the sedating effects of alcohol, a narcotic drug. As little as two drinks of alcohol impairs judgement (the reasoning – and spiritual-discernment centres of the brain) and weakens one's self-control. Caffeine, a true stimulant drug, can produce reactions in the body which are indistinguishable from those of an anxiety attack – such as dizziness, sleep difficulties and recurring headaches. Caffeine causes a rise in fat and glucose in the blood stream, thereby encouraging fat storage in the body. Avoid "diet" or artificially sweetened carbonated beverages as no study has shown that they have any weight control benefit. If anything, they promote cravings.

10. Avoid TV viewing and reading magazines that contain tempting advertisements of unhealthful foods. Keep busy on a pleasant, useful program.

11. Remember that the Bible is a veritable gold mine of promises of Divine help for all difficult situations. The following texts are but a few of them. I would challenge

you to discover more through your personal Bible study and make them your own.

Matthew 7:7-11
God is more willing to give good things to those that ask Him than parents are willing to give good gifts to their children.

Romans 12:1-2
We are to present our bodies to God for His service in the best possible condition.

1 Corinthians 3:16, 17 and 6:19, 20
Keeping our bodies in the very best health possible is a means of glorifying God.

1 Corinthians 10:13
God never allows temptation to be greater than we can bear.

Galatians 6:9
We are not to grow discouraged in the work of forming correct habits – for in due time we shall see the benefits of our efforts and prayers.

Philippians 1:6
God is able to complete the good work that He begins in us.

Philippians 4:13
We can do all things through Christ who is our strength.

3 John 2
God desires both our body and soul to be healthy.

Jude 24
God is able to keep us from falling (into temptation).

When we try to separate ourselves from unhealthful habits, it may seem at times that we are tearing ourselves apart. But it is the very work we must do if we would grow up into the full stature of men and women in Christ. That point where known duty crosses personal inclination is the very point where God's power can manifest itself in our life. Jesus said that without Him, we can do nothing; but with Him, we can do everything (John 15:5)

When we choose to put into practice good eating habits and healthful lifestyle – even though it may go against every inclination or clamouring of our nature – God's power is available to put into action that choice we have made.

The effort we put into carrying out our good choices is the tangible manifestation of God's power in our experience. The action is ours – the power is God's. The action requires effort from every part of our being – our nerves, muscles and mental concentration. It is encouraging to know that with watchfulness and prayer, our weakest point and most difficult temptation can be so guarded as to become our character strength or strongest point.

References

Clinical Guidelines on the Identification, Evaluation, and Treatment of Overweight and Obesity in Aducts. National Institutes of Health, National Heart, Lung and Blood Institute, June 1998

www.niddk.nih.gov/health/nutrit/pubs/statobes.htm#what

www.cnn.com/HEALTH/library/DS/00314.html

www.who.int/dietphysicalactivity/publications/facts/obesity/en/

The Press, Christchurch, New Zealand, Aug 21, 2004

Natural Lifestyle and your Health Magazine – by Mary Ann Kimmel-McNeilus, MD

Sugar: The Sweet Mystery of Life

Years ago when I was taking voice lessons, I learned of a song with the opening line, "Ah, Sweet Mystery of Life, at last I've found you!" Back then I thought that referred to snickers and moro bars!

How I loved my sweets and lollies, not to mention the ice creams, biscuits and pies and anything else that contained that "sweet mystery of life". It was only a few years ago that I realized that sugar was NOT the sweet mystery of life, but rather a most unsuspected precursor of disease and death.

Facing the Problem

I was raised in a family that believed sugar and children grew together like flowers and sunshine. Only now, after years of suffering the consequences of that philosophy, do I realise that the children need a **lot** of things, but **not** generous amounts of sugar. As flowers wilt with too much sunshine and not enough water, eventually children (and adults) will wilt from large quantities of sugar, especially as these sugary foods crowd out adequate amounts of other vital nutrients.

As I grew older, my sugar habit began to cause me considerable trouble. I was not well much most of the time and when I was "well", I still didn't feel good. I had to come to the point of admitting that I had a problem. How was I to solve it?

I tried not eating any sugar for a while, but the yearning for sweets or doughnuts was more overpowering than I could bear. I just **had** to have my "fix" of sugar.

I did not realise until recently the powerful bondage sugar had put me in. I was a *sugarholic* and needed to do something about it. Like a dependent alcoholic, I was enslaved in a health destroying habit; sugar was my master.

I talked the problem over with several friends, but no one seemed to sense the seriousness of my situation. When I talked about my sugar cravings and addiction, they would say, "Just don't eat it any more if it bothers you." Or, "It's not that bad for you as long as you keep in in moderation."

Easier said than done! And besides, who stipulates moderation?

It was only when I started reading and researching on foods and nutrition that I realised how victimised I was by the sugar in my lifestyle. The detrimental effects sugar has on the body are serious, but not more serious that its captivating control. How was I to get free?

It was not until I admitted my problem to the Lord and asked for victory over this overpowering influence that I began to wean away from its deadly grips. Notice I said "wean" away. It was not an overnight victory.

Sugar Addiction

What caused this addiction to sugar? Where did it come from? How can it play such a major role in our daily lives and just how harmful is it? How can we change our taste buds to desire the non-sugared foods?

For one thing, we must decide to completely change. Just cutting down doesn't work. I found in my own life that the more sugar you eat, the more sugar you want, and even when you think you are tapering off, if you put sugar into the body, the cravings will continue. If you remove all sugar and persist in keeping it out of your diet, the cravings subside until they are finally subdued.

In addition, our taste buds have been altered over the past 90 years to such an extent that we have, to a degree, lost the taste for natural, good, nutritious foods. I have watched people put sugar on watermelon and peaches because they don't taste sweet enough.

If our taste buds weren't so perverted, we could really enjoy the natural sweets the way God intended them to be enjoyed.

How Much Sugar Do We Eat?

By the early 1900's, on the average, every man, woman and child in the United States, was eating approximately 20 kg of sugar per year. Today estimates range from 45 kg to 100 kg per year.

Do you know how much sugar 20 kg per year is? Divided into a daily portion, it is 27 teaspoonful per day. Where are we getting that much? In reality, it isn't very hard to reach that level of intake and greatly exceed it.

Consider the following chart of hidden sugars in common "Western" foods:

Hidden Sugars in Foods

Foods	Portion Size	Sugar Content (approx. tsp.)
Fruit Pie	1 slice	10
Chocolate Cake	1 piece	10
Glazed doughnut	1	6
Soft Drinks	250 mL glass	5
Chocolates	30g	4
Ice Cream	1 scoop	4
Canned Fruit	1 serving	3
Jellies and Jams	1 Tablespoon	3
Canned vegetables and beans	1 serving	2-3

In some ways we are eating less sugar than we used to consume. The household use of sugar has dropped to half of what it was in the early 1900's and total sweets consumption is down from what was consumed in the 1940's, yet the total sugar consumption is steadily on the rise. How can this be?

The food processing corporations are utilising sugar in just about everything we eat, and most of us don't realise it because we don't take time to read the labels.

Do you know where you are getting sugar? Consider these points:
- There is more sugar poured into processed fruits and vegetables and desserts now than ever before
- The soft drink industry has increased its varieties, thereby encouraging greater consumption of sweetened soft drinks.
- The cereal industry advocates the importance of all the vitamins and minerals in their cereals, but fail to note the addition of up to three times more sugar than when they originally started creating their product.

The sweet things are not the only "foods" that increase our intake of sugar. Junk foods that we would never classify as "sweets" cause us serious sugar problems as well. So-called "foods" such as corn chips, potato chips, etc. are refined carbohydrates which are turned into simple sugars in the mouth then dumped into the digestive system.

These "non-sweet" snacks have almost as much tendency to raise blood sugar levels as do cakes and biscuits. They also have just about as much tendency to cause tooth decay as sugar does. The enzyme, Ptyalin, produced by the salivary gland in the mouth, converts starches to sugar as you chew. During digestion, starch (long chains of sugar molecules) are broken down into sugar and will have an effect similar to sugar.

When sugar is the second or third ingredient on the label, you know it's way too much. As far as the body is concerned, sugar is sugar from whatever source.

Learning Young
Where are our children learning to consume so many sweets?

It doesn't take much observation to figure that out.

From Mums: I once read that the mother is the primary person who moulds the child's taste buds. Unfortunately, too many mothers think that children need sweets and they use these treats for incentives and rewards.

From TV: Have you noticed the kinds of advertisements that come on during the hours when children are normally watching TV? Sweetened cereals, chewing gums, soft drinks, biscuits and junk foods in general! Unfortunately children now grow up with the television and it has become one of their primary educators.

Advertisements are **not** harmless? They are very subtle influences in the "spongy" minds of innocent children. Children don't know what is best for their diet unless they are educated. Parents have a great responsibility to educate their children in correct and healthy habits.

Other Advertising: Advertisers are not stupid. Children have a powerful influence on the grocery buyer of the family. Designers are well aware of the power children have to play on their parents' emotions while in the supermarkets and shops.

Why so Much Concern Over Sugar?
So what harm does a little sweet treat or junk food do to the body? Plenty! Many diseases are directly attributed to high sugar intake. Eighty percent of all other countries in the world do not show the chronic disease which the western world exhibits today. The "developed" countries, USA, Europe, Australia, and New Zealand, show a direct correlation between the increase and the amount of sugar consumed and increase of diseases.

Diseases: Throat infections, colds, sinus problems and yeast infections are especially prominent in doctor's offices following

Christmas and Easter. Excess sugar utilises important B and C vitamins which are necessary for the immune system.

Other diseases aggravated by sugar are Asthma, mental illness, and nervous disorders. B vitamins are needed to coat the nerves and keep them healthy. Excess sugar utilised the important B vitamins for metabolisation of the sugar and strips the nerves of their protective coating, causing irritability.

Two other major diseases affected by an excess of sugar in the system are **diabetes** and **heart disease**. We have seen a prominent rise in these two diseases over the last fifty years and it's scary. They are not known in eighty percent of other countries **and** are preventable.

Sugar causes a rise in blood pressure and creates an imbalance of the calcium/phosphorus ration which directly affects the heart. It also causes the pancreas to produce more insulin as the blood sugar level increases. Remember that fats more directly affect the blood sugar level than sugar, but the combination of the two is deadly.

Eyes: Did you know that you may be wearing glasses needlessly? Near sightedness and the amount of refined carbohydrates in the diet have been found to be almost directly proportional.

Constipation: Sugar, along with a lack of fibre, insufficient water in the diet, and the high fat content of foods, causes constipation – chronic or acute sluggishness of the bowl. Constipation is more a chronic problem now than ever before, yielding the laxative industry over $200 million per year.

Your Teeth: Half of all Americans have no teeth at all by the time they reach the age of fifty-five. It is now known that sugar, which is chewed in one form or another, coats the teeth and tends to slow down or stop the individual circulation system of each tooth. As circulation is hindered, the normal streptococcus bacteria, which is always in the mouth, mixes with the sugar and causes decay. If you can't brush immediately after a meal to clean the sugars off your teeth, your mouth should at least be rinsed thoroughly with water within fifteen minutes.

Remember, **"If you are not true to your teeth, they will be false to you"**.

Overeating and Diet: The diet industry is another multi-million dollar industry which has taken advantage of the western sweet tooth. There is no doubt that excess sugar yields excess calories which are devoid of nutrition. Excess calories yield excess weight.

Behavior: Notice how your children act within an hour after eating an excess of sugar and junk food. Notice yourself how you feel after a heavy dessert. There have been definite personality changes and mood swings observed.

So What Good is Sugar?
Why do we continue to eat so much sugar when we know it harms our minds and bodies? How can we alter our taste buds to enjoy other more nutritional foods?

Energy Sources
We have been told by the advertisers of candy bars that sugar is energy and is needed for a quick "picker-upper". Unfortunately too many people believe that.

Complex carbohydrates are the true source of energy without all the side effects of sugar. We must realise that the more sugar we eat, the more we want. Likewise, the less we eat, the less we want.

Alternatives
The Lord gave us a natural sweetener to use – honey. But even then He instructed us not to eat too much of it. *"Have you found*

honey? Eat only what you need, let you have it in excess and vomit it". (Proverbs 25:16)

Other alternatives are: malt, molasses, fruit juice, dried fruits (especially dates) and fresh or canned fruits.

Making a Change
In order to realise a change in our lifestyle we must first come to grips with ourselves and admit to our addictions, sugar being of an addictive nature. Remember that of ourselves we can do nothing *"but with God all things are possible". (Matthew 19:26)*

Some of the things that work with me, which have worked with many others, are:
1. **Don't by any more sweets.** If they are not around they won't be a temptation.
2. **Gradually adjust your taste buds** to enjoy the more natural tasting sweets, such as dates, raisins, apples, peaches, etc.
3. **As you eat less artificial sweets, the natural will taste sweeter.** It takes approximately 300 mm of sugar cane to produce 5-7 teaspoons of sugar.
4. **Be aware of the sugar content in the foods you eat. READ LABELS!** Remember that all processed foods contain sugar. Words ending with *-ose* are sugars (such as dextrose, sucrose, fructose, etc.).
5. **Remember that rich desserts are poor in nutrients.** Although enjoyable, they are deplorable to the body and should be avoided.
6. **Have a support system,** someone to "kick the habit" with, preferably your family.
7. **Break the *dessert thinking*.** It's ingrained in us to have something sweet after a good meal. Satisfy that desire by ending your meal with a good tooth brushing. The freshness in the mouth will satisfy the desire of the sweet craving.
8. **Drink plenty of water.** Often the craving for something sweet is the body's way of saying "I'm thirsty!" but don't

drink with the meals. Use water up to half an hour before a meal and at least an hour and a half after a meal.

9. When the temptation for a goodie becomes overwhelming, remember that the Lord is there to help you. Don't try to overcome it on your own, but ask Him for help.

"Wherefore let him that thinketh he standeth take heed lest he fall. There hath no temptation taken you but such as is common to man: but God is faithful, who will not suffer you to be tempted above that ye are able; but will with the temptation also make a way to escape, that ye may be able to bear it." (1 Corinthians 10:12, 13)

Knowing that what you eat affects your mind, and knowing that sugar has a tendency to dull the senses and cloud the thinking and understanding, that we can only hear God speaking if our minds are clear, *"then whatever you eat or drink or whatever you do, do all to the glory of God". (1 Corinthians 10:31)*

You will gain complete victory over any sugar habit by following the simple natural diet God outlined for us in the beginning – Fruits, Nuts, Grains and Vegetables (Gen. 1:29; 3:18)

Taken from *Natural Lifestyle and your Health* magazine – by Nancy Riedestel

Diabetes:
Sweet Tooth, Bitter Harvest

She called the Lifestyle Centre of America, desperate for help. Thirty years of diabetes had taken its tremendous toil on her health. The high blood sugars had done their work silently for years, but now the bitter harvest was undeniably obvious. Jenny had kidney failure and resulting fluid accumulation. Of more concern to her, however, was that she was going blind. Her vision had been getting progressively worse, and the doctors had given her no hope. With these discouraging prospects ahead she became excited as she heard about a lifestyle approach toward reversing the effects of diabetes.

This report comes from America, but there are so many similar cases, especially in the western world. Tragically though, it often takes irreversible complications before people really get serious about doing all they can to control their diabetes. By then it is too late to accomplish all that is humanly possible to reverse the case that could have been helped if only treatment could have been started earlier. Many newly diagnosed diabetics, as well as those struggling with the disease for longer periods of time, can control their diabetes without drugs by following an excellent lifestyle. Do not wait until a heart attack, or amputation, or blindness serves as a wake-up call. The wake-up call should be the first "border-line blood sugar" – the slightest suggestion of diabetes.

What exactly is Diabetes?
Diabetes mellitus or "sugar diabetes" is a condition where an abnormal response to insulin and/or inadequate insulin production causes high blood sugar levels. This is usually defined by a fasting blood sugar of greater than 125 on two occasions or a positive glucose tolerance test (the individual drinks a specified amount of glucose, usually 75 grams, and their blood sugars are evaluated over a two hour period). Over time, these high blood sugar levels

and the other metabolic changes that go along with diabetes, are extremely taxing on the body. Consequently, diabetes dramatically increases ones risk of death and disability.

Current statistics are sobering. In America there are now three times as many diabetics as there were in 1958. Estimates are that some 16 million Americans now have this condition, up from 11 million as recent as 1983. Depending on the type of diabetics and other characteristics, they run anywhere from 2-12 times the risk of death when compared to their non-diabetic peers.

Although heart disease is the leading cause of death among diabetics, sometimes the debilitating effects of blindness and kidney disease are more frightening.

Within only seven years of diagnosis, as many as 50 percent of children with diabetes have developed diabetic retinopathy, a disease of the eyes that can result in blindness. Diabetics need to be checked by eye doctors regularly. Diabetic eye disease is preventable, not only through lifestyle, but also by early treatment. Furthermore, diabetics run a significant risk of developing kidney disease. In any given year, some 55,000 Americans are suffering with what is called "end-stage renal disease" due to their diabetes.

All Diabetics are not the same

Diabetics are often divided into four categories. Of these four categories, there are actually two main types of diabetes: insulin-dependent diabetes mellitus (IDDM), often referred to as Type I, and non-insulin dependent diabetes mellitus (NIDDM), often designated as Type II.

Type I diabetes is the most severe form of the disease. It typically occurs in childhood (but can develop at any age) and for this reason was previously called "juvenile diabetes". The most common cause of Type I diabetes is destruction of the insulin-making cells in the pancreas by the person's own immune system. This is referred to as "autoimmune destruction". The specific factors that trigger this autoimmune process have proved elusive. Although some cases have been linked to viruses or chemical toxins, much is still unknown about the beginning of the Type I diabetes process. There does seem to be a genetic susceptibility to the disease, plus an environmental factor that triggers the diseases process. Some of the most interesting recent research links some cases of Type I diabetes to an abnormal immune reaction to milk protein. We now know that children who are breast fed for a shorter time or who are started on cow's milk earlier have an increased risk for this type of diabetes. In fact, the drinking of cow's milk may be the trigger that initiates the disease in over half of all Type I diabetics.

Regardless of the cause of their Type I diabetes, affected individual lose their ability to make adequate amounts of insulin and are left with an absolute life-and-death need for insulin shots. Without those shots, they go into a condition called diabetic ketoacidosis, which is fatal if not promptly treated. Because of their absolute need for insulin, individuals with Type I diabetes are usually diagnosed early in the disease process.

The main fuel for our bodies is a simple sugar called glucose. There is a potential problem, however, with this fuel source. It can only get into each cell of the body if insulin is present. Some have compared insulin to a key that opens "the doors" in the body cells so that the vital fuel, glucose, can get into the cell. However, if there is an insufficient amount of insulin (as in Type I diabetes) or if the lock on the doors are "gummed up" so that the insulin key has difficulty opening them (as can occur with the insulin resistance of Type II diabetes), then blood sugar levels can rise. When blood sugar levels rise sufficiently, the ability of the kidneys to contain the sugar is overwhelmed, and sugar comes out in the urine. The sugar takes water with it, thus leading to the excessive urination so familiar in uncontrolled diabetes. The loss of water results in another diabetes symptom: increased thirst. At the same time, sugar is not moving into the body's cells adequately. In a sense, the body's cells are starving for energy. This can cause fatigue, weight loss, and excessive hunger.

Fortunately, only about 5-10 percent of diabetics in America fall under the Type I diabetes category. The remainder are Type II diabetics.

Many individuals with Type II diabetes generate plenty of insulin but their body is resistant to it. This condition of insulin resistance can be addressed by lifestyle changes. By maintaining an excellent diet, achieving an ideal weight, and embarking on an exercise programme, many Type II diabetics can control their blood sugars with their lifestyle changes along. Some may need diet changes plus a pill to help control their blood sugar.

Because of the more subtle nature of Type II diabetes compared to Type I, it often goes undiagnosed. A person with Type II diabetes may not have any of the classic diabetes signs, like excessive urination, excessive thirst, excessive hunger, fatigue or weight loss. At any point in time, it is estimated that fully 50 percent of Type II diabetics have not yet been diagnosed. Of course, unrecognised diabetes still does its damage steadily and silently. Even about 20 percent of newly diagnosed Type II diabetics already had damage to their eyes (retinopathy).

Although Type II diabetes can be picked up by such blood tests for elevated sugar, many people do not seek health professional for such preventative services. They wait until they are sick. This is unfortunate. As a result, Type II diabetics only become aware of their disease when they experience potentially irreversible problems like eye or kidney disease, nerve problems or a heart attack.

Diabetes in the unborn
Regarding gestational diabetes, 2-5 percent of all pregnant American women are affected. This translates into about 200,000

children being born to mothers with gestational diabetes each year. This is significant, because those children experience an increased risk of health disorders such as birth trauma, lower blood sugars at birth (neonatal hypoglycemia) and even premature death in infancy (prenatal mortality). The message is clear: if you are a diabetic who becomes pregnant, or if you develop gestational diabetes, you should have your blood sugar monitored closely. Your diet and lifestyle need to be well regulated. Furthermore, any woman who develops gestational diabetes has a genetic tendency for diabetes. She is at high risk to develop full-blown diabetes later in life. Practising healthy habits throughout her life span thus becomes critical.

Controlling Diabetes
Recently, a landmark Diabetes Control and complication Trial was completed. This six-year study looked at 1441 Type 1 juvenile diabetics. Those diabetics who strove to keep their blood sugar as close to normal as possible (using insulin and lifestyle changes) had 76 percent less chance of developing diabetic retinopathy (eye disease). They also experienced fewer cases of significant kidney disease and 60 percent fewer cases of nerve problems involving the hands and/or feet (peripheral neuropathy). The participants also significantly lowered their blood cholesterol levels, suggesting that tight control could decrease heart disease risk by up to 35 percent.

For Type II diabetics, although they are non-insulin dependent, this simply means that they do don have a life or death need for insulin shots. Many doctors nonetheless put these individuals on insulin to better control their blood sugars. In fact, the National Institutes of Health indicate that 50 percent of known Type II diabetics in America are either using insulin alone or insulin in combination with oral medications. This greatly confuses many in lay circles. They erroneously think that just because someone is on insulin, they are a Type I diabetic. More often than not, a diabetic who is on insulin has the Type II variety.

According to Dr. Neil Nedley, M.D. researcher in Cardiology, Gastroenterology, Critical Care and Preventative Medicine, based on published medical research and personal experience, states that careful blood sugar control is important in Type II diabetics. However, the use of insulin and oral agents in these individuals carries the potential to do more harm than good. Thus, the most important question in his mind always is: how can he help his Type II diabetic patients control their sugars without drugs? Such an approach stands to reduce the complications of high blood sugars while decreasing the risk of problems from treatment.

Non-Drug Approach brings startling results

Many seem to think that using a non-drug approach would increase the risk of diabetic complications and decrease the likelihood of attaining optimal blood sugar control. Ironically, the evidence suggests that the opposite is true: an optimal lifestyle programme sees to help many diabetics more than any drugs available. One recent example of the power of a comprehensive lifestyle programme comes from Weimar Institute in California. Researchers there studied the benefits of a live-in, 25-day comprehensive lifestyle programme on Type II diabetic patients. A frequent complication of diabetes is peripheral neuropathy, a condition that often manifests itself as burning or aching sensations in the feet and legs and may also involve the hands and arms. The pain is often described as excruciating and sharp. The disease can later progress to numbness, as heat, cold and pain can no longer be felt in the affected areas. Although medications may sometimes help the condition, they often make no significant impact.

The study's lead researcher was Dr. Milton Crate (an endocrinologist who specialises in reversing the effect of diabetes through lifestyle changes). He showed that a meatless diet, free from all animal products and high in unrefined total vegetarian foods, will bring complete relief to painful neuropathy in over 80 percent of diabetics with this condition in just 4-16 days.

Other elements of the programme included: regular exercise, hydrotherapy treatments, cooking classes, group lectures, exclusion of a variety of beverages (coffee, tea, and alcohol), exclusion of tobacco, and for those who desired, religious counselling.

Previously, diabetic neuropathy was thought to be incurable. This study shows that the condition can actually be reversed through a comprehensive lifestyle programme that includes diet and exercise. Blood sugars and cholesterol dramatically improved on this diet. The benefits of complete relief of diabetic painful neuropathy continue according to a one to four year follow-up programme.

Exercise
Exercise plays a powerful role in lowering blood sugar levels. Evidence suggests that muscles in motion reduce resistance to insulin; that is, insulin sensitivity is improved by regular exercise. More simply put, exercise – in a sense – works like insulin in a diabetic: it helps sugar go out of the blood and into the muscle tissue. In fact, the prestigious Joslin's Diabetic Medical textbook indicates that lack of exercise is a "key factor" in the development of insulin resistance, as people get older. Since diabetics need insulin on a daily basis (either their own body's insulin or injected insulin), so do diabetics need daily exercise to optimally control their blood sugars and their disease.

Proper Diet
Until recently, diabetics were told that in order to control their blood sugars they had to eliminate most of the carbohydrates from their diet. They were told to avoid sugar, but the message did not stop there. Plant foods – naturally rich in complex carbohydrates – were also on the "hit list". The results left diabetics gravitating to a heavy meat diet. With heavy meat consumption also came increased ingestion of cholesterol and saturated fat. Galloping atherosclerosis then followed close behind.

Notwithstanding the fact that meat can help control blood sugars in diabetics, a large Southern Californian study done among Seventh-Day Adventists showed that those that ate meat six or more times per week were at 3.8 times greater risk of dying from diabetes than those who ate meat less than once per week. Other research indicates an additional benefit to diabetics who avoid meat and animal products. These animal derived items have no fibre in them whatsoever. Fibre is emerging as a critical ingredient in blood sugar control. In fact, some suggest that an abundant supply of fibre is one of the main reasons that a vegetarian diet benefits diabetics.

Fibre facts
Fibre is a term that refers to plant constituents that are resistant to human digestive enzymes. It is generally classified as either soluble (dissolves in water) or insoluble, both essential for good nutrition, especially in diabetics. One of the bonuses of eating a balanced diet of natural plant foods is that we tend to get liberal amounts of both the soluble and insoluble fibres.

Research makes evident that foods that are high in fibre lead to a slower rise in blood sugar and as a result, require less insulin to handle the meal. Fibre, especially soluble fibre like pectin and gums, slows the emptying of food from the stomach and helps to slow the absorption of simple sugars in the small intestine. This should be contrasted with high fat meals that can result in high blood glucose levels for up to five hours after the meal.
Dr. James Anderson and colleagues at the University of Kentucky found that by using a high carbohydrate and high fibre diet, the need for insulin was greatly reduced. Blood sugar control was better and fasting levels of cholesterol and triglycerides fell.

Many nutrition experts recommend that our diet should contain between 20-35 grams of fibre per day when it comes to issues like cancer prevention. However, even higher amounts of fibre seem optimal for diabetes control

Consumption of soluble fibre also appears to be important in non-diabetics. As we have already noted, whether or not a person has diabetes, these fibres prevent the rapid rise in blood sugar, with a resulting lower peak level. Therefore, insulin requirements are actually decreased when these fibres are added to the diet. This is no small matter. As important as insulin is in controlling our blood sugar, ongoing research demonstrates that higher blood insulin levels increase the speed at which the blockages of atherosclerosis develop. Thus, we should help our bodies by placing fewer demands of high insulin output. One way we can do this is by eating less sugar and choosing more fibre rich foods.

Conclusion

Dr. Neil Nedley concludes by adding "many of my diabetic patients request that I give them a very specific menu that will help control their diabetes. However, for most diabetics, menus are not as important as knowing and practising the dietary *principles* of diabetic control. This is especially true for the non-insulin dependent Type II diabetic. The principles are really very basic. The more natural fruits, vegetables, and whole grains the better (nuts are also good in moderation). The less meat and dairy products the better. The less refined sugar the better. The more fibre the better. Eat a good breakfast and little, if any evening meal. If you are overweight, it is of utmost importance that you reduce your weight to your ideal (thus the less fat in the diet the better) and follow an eating style that allows you to attain and maintain this reasonable weight.

"Do not feel bound to some restrictive way of eating. Take the principles to heart. Experiment with different options. You will be surprised at how enjoyable a healthy lifestyle can really be."

-Taken from the book "Proof Positive", chapter eight "Sweet Tooth, Bitter Harvest", by Dr. Neil Nedley M.D., full time practicing physician in Internal Medicine with emphasis in Cardiology, Gastroenterology, Critial Care, and Preventative Medicine.

THE MIRACLE OF
ONIONS AND GARLIC

Garlic and onions are very good for the entire body. They have similar qualities that are extremely helpful in many situations. Listed below are some of the ways they will benefit the system.

- Thins the blood
- Retards blood clotting
- Lowers blood sugar
- Kills bacteria
- Relieves bronchial congestion
- Blocks cancer
- Fights colds
- Lowers blood pressure
- Heart tonic
- Diuretic
- Purifies blood
- Expectorants (promotes secretion from Mucus membranes)
- Relieves coughs
- Aids insomnia
- Raises the immunological functions

HOW MUCH TO USE

1. Half a raw onion a day can boost your good HDL blood cholesterol by an average of 30%.
2. A tablespoon of cooked onions will lower the clotting tendency of the blood thus reducing the chance of a stroke.
3. Half a cup of onions raw or cooked can clean your blood, thus keeping the blood in great shape.
4. One cup of onion juice a week keeps the blood in better shape to fend off cardiovascular disease.
5. Two ounces of onion juice per day will lower your blood pressure.

ONIONS

George Washington said: "My remedy is always to eat, just before I step into bed, a hot roasted onion, if I have a cold."

Onions have a very sensitive organism and absorb all morbid matter. If you place an onion in a sick room where infection is in the air, the onion will become very dark or black as it absorbs the poisonous matter.

An onion will not only kill an infection, but will also lower blood pressure, stimulate the lungs, skin, etc., aid the digestive juices, help hoarseness and an inflamed throat.

A roasted onion is very good for earaches, a sore throat, and a sore chest while garlic and onion combined are beneficial for a toothache.

ANTI-ASTHMATIC ONION
Onions, from the same family as garlic, possess anti-asthmatic properties. The onion's action in relieving asthma is due to its ability to inhibit the production of compounds which cause the bronchial muscle to spasm along with its ability to relax the bronchial muscle. Place a bowl of sliced or chopped onions by your bed. Breathing the fumes of the onion will help open up and purify the sinuses.

BLADDER INFECTION
Take the juice of 3 onions, 3 radishes and 5 lemons. Mix and take 1 tsp. 5 times daily (see the end of this section for how to juice).

BLOOD SUGAR LEVELS
The onion has been shown in tests to have a hypoglycemic effect. Onion extracts from dried onions were given and greatly lowered the blood sugar levels. Thus those with diabetes would realty benefit by daily consumption of onions.

BOILS
Boil onions until soft, or if raw, mash to a pulp and add vegetable oil to keep them from hardening. Spread this mixture on a cloth and apply to the boil. This is also simulating to sluggish or slow sores.

CANCER PREVENTION
Onions consist of concentrated substances that contain sulphur and can turn off cell changes that lead to cancer growth. Just one-half cup of onions per day, raw or cooked, may boost your cancer-prevention quotient.

CHILDREN WITH WORMS
Cut up two raw onions and let them soak for 24 hours in one quart of distilled water. Strain and teaspoon the juice to the child throughout the day. A little water may be added to dilute the taste. Honey may be added if necessary to make the taste palatable. This should be used with an enema, made from equal parts of plantain and catnip, and black walnut in the proper dose.

CHOLESTEROL LEVELS BALANCED
Dr. Gurewich, Professor of Medicine at Tufts University has identified some 150 compounds in onions, all of which are involved in increasing HDL levels by about 30% while decreasing LDL levels. A one-half medium sized onion per day is sufficient to produce these results.

COLD CONGESTION
Steam some onions in a frying pan in a little water and then thicken with corn starch. Apply to the chest in a pillow case and cover with a heating pad.

COUGH SYRUP
To make a cough syrup, stir one pint of chopped onion in one half cup of honey and add ½ tsp. cayenne pepper. Keep the mixture

warm by placing in hot water or a warm place. Take 1 tsp. as needed.

DISINFECTING WOUNDS
Chopped, diced, or squeezed for its juice, the onion disinfects the wound. Mix the onion with apple cider vinegar and apply to the wound (see the end of this section for how to juice).

DRAWING POULTICE
Potatoes, like onions, draw infection and impurities from the body. Blend up or chop 2 potatoes and 3 onions. Make a poultice by placing this mixture in gauze and putting it on the infection or put directly on the skin, drawing out the heat and infection.

DRY EYES
For congested or dry eyes, peel and chop onions so that the tea duct opens.

EARACHE/EAR INFECTION
Cut an onion in half, bake it for 5 minutes, then cool and tie over the ear. This will give relief when pain is severe, and it also has antibiotic properties (See earache under garlic section).

FINGERNAILS AND TOENAILS
Brittle finger or toenails can be improved by rubbing the juice of an onion several times a day. You may cut an onion and rub the juice directly on the nails or juice the onion and use the juice throughout the day (see the end of this section for how to juice).

GOUT
Make a raw onion poultice by chopping or grating the onion and put it over the affected area. Leave it on all night.

HEMORRHOIDS
It has been reported that eating cooked onions will stop the bleeding and pain of hemorrhoids. A person reported that when

the onions were eaten, there was no bleeding, but on the days when the onions were eliminated from the diet, the bleeding occurred.

HOT POTATO AND ONION, INHALATION
For congestion, particularly sinus congestion, inhale the steam of boiled potatoes and onions. Continue this treatment until the potatoes cool and the steam has stopped. Pine needles and onions boiled are even more effective.

HICCUPS
A fast remedy for this problem is to take a tablespoon of raw onion juice every one-half hour (see the end of this section for how to juice).

HIGH IN MINERAL, SILICA
Onions are one food that has a very high content of silica. Silica is a mineral that has a direct connection with the absorption of all minerals. This mineral is imperative for the elasticity of the lung tissue and its function. It also helps in skin disorders, injuries, bone diseases, diseases of the intestinal tract, urinary disorders, and bleeding gums.

INFLUENZA
Take two chopped garlic bulbs and three chopped onion bulbs and place in a blender and blend with a small amount of water. Add 3 Tbsp of olive oil to this mixture. Give 1 Tbsp as needed.

LUNG INFECTION
Boil onions, mash them and place them between two layers of cloth. Apply to the chest for about two hours.

NERVES AND MENTAL FATIGUE
Onions are a good source of silicon which is necessary for healthy nerves and to reduce mental fatigue. Include them in the diet daily.

NOSEBLEEDS OR BLEEDING GUMS

Take the juice of an onion and mix with apple cider vinegar. This solution may be used for nose bleeding by snuffing drop up the nose with an eye-dropper. You may also hold the same solution in the mouth for bleeding gums (see the end of this section for how to juice).

STY

Chop onions to cause the eyes to tear. Thus, eyes will be moistened and drained. You can also place a nice sized slice of onion (for only a few minutes) over the closed eye with the sty to draw out the infection. Gently wash off the area where the onion was laying.

GARLIC

Garlic has been used throughout history for the treatment of a wide variety of conditions. Sanskrit records document the use of garlic remedies approximately 5,000 years ago, while the Chinese have been using it for at least 3,000 years. The Codex Ebers, an Egyptian medical papyrus dating to about 1550 B.C., mentions garlic as an effective remedy for a long list of ailments. In general, garlic has been used as a medicine throughout the world for a very long time.

ANEMIA
In one study, after eight weeks of a treatment with garlic extract or cooked garlic (best to use raw in anemia), there was shown a very nice improvement in the hemoglobin.

ANTIBIOTIC TEA – ONION AND GRAPEFRUIT
Cut up 2 grapefruits, 3 onion bulbs, 2 garlic bulbs, 6 lemons with peeling and put in 1 ½ quarts of water. Add 1 cup of peach leaf or yarrow tea and let simmer for 3-5 minutes; cool. Drink ½ cup every hour for 5-6 hours.

ANTIOXIDANT QUALITIES
Garlic is high in selenium which acts as an antioxidant. It converts the free radicals into less reactive and harmful forms. This prevents the accumulation of free radicals.

ARTHRITIS
Dr. Jack Soltanoff of West Hurley, New York, reports that garlic is very helpful in arthritic pain relief. He states that one clove daily may be chewed and swallowed. It may also be chopped fine and stirred into a salad or sprinkle on other foods.

For a painful joint, peel two large heads of garlic, chop and soak in one-half cup of warm olive oil for five minutes. Dip a thick sock in hot water and wring out the excess water. Fill the toe with the garlic/olive oil mixture and rub it over the painful joint for 3-5 minutes.

A Rusk Institute of New York therapist, Barry Ostrow, suggests wrapping diced garlic in a hot damp washcloth and rubbing the painful area for 15-20 minutes. For those who prefer cold to hot applications, the garlic may be placed in a damp washcloth and frozen. Joint pain of a new onset may be treated with the application of the cold garlic pack for ten minutes every two hours for the first 36 hours. Chronic pain may be treated with ten to twenty minute hot applications two or three times a day.

BLADDER –IRRITATION OF
The best remedy for any bladder irritation was considered to be corn-silk, onion and garlic. Take ½ cup of corn-silk, 3 onions and 2 quarts of water and make a tea. Drink 2-3 cups of this tea daily.

BLOOD CLOTS
Both onion and garlic contain substances that inhibit platelet aggregation. Prior to a blood clot forming, platelets clump together to help in the development of the clot. Garlic and onions should be included in the diet daily to reduce the risk of blood clots. They may be eaten, raw or cooked, as the factor which reduces platelet stickiness is stable after heating.

CARDIOVASCULAR SYSTEM IMPROVES
Garlic oil is beneficial for the heart and cardiovascular system (see the recipe for garlic oil). This oil may be used in many ways including in salad dressings. Also, 1 Tbsp a day may be taken. If this leaves a strong odour, chew on parsley to eliminate it.

COLDS, ETC.
Onion and garlic tea: Cut three large onions and two bulbs or garlic. Place in one and a half quarts or water and saute until tender. Add ½ tsp. cayenne pepper. Drink 2 oz every hour for 5-6 hours.

TEA FOR CHILDREN

Garlic has excellent antibiotic properties, but your child will probably detest the taste of it. A tea made of lemon and garlic will overcome this problem. Cut a garlic clove into small pieces and mash with the bowl of a spoon. Place one teaspoon of peppermint or mint in a teapot, add the mashed garlic and the juice of ¼ of a lemon. Add boiling water and steep for about 5 minutes. Strain and serve. Drink one cup three times daily.

In the book *Healing Power of Garlic* (see the Reference Section), the author gives his favorite cold treatment: "Blend three garlic cloves in ½ cup of carrot juice and swallow the whole thing down. Do this three times a day. Make a soup of garlic, onions and greens and have that in place of a meal."

CORNS

"Crush equal amounts of garlic and onions into a paste. Clean the area round the corn and disinfect it with alcohol. Trim it down with a knife as far as possible but not deep enough to make it bleed. Soak the food in salt water. In about twenty minutes, the corn becomes soft. Moisten the garlic/onion paste with vinegar. Put this directly on the corn and cover it with a bandage. Leave it on for 20 minutes. Repeat the process every other day. The corn will usually heal within a week." (Section from the book *The Healing Power of Garlic*. See the Reference Section).

DETOX – CLEAN OUT TOXINS

Chop or juice the onions or garlic. Take 1 tsp of this every hour during the day. The chopped onion or juice may be mixed with catnip tea, sage tea or honey (see the end of this section for how to juice).

DIGESTIVE DISORDERS

Crushed cloves of garlic may be infused in water and taken for all disorders of the digestion. To infuse garlic, crush one ounce of garlic and pour one pint of boiling water over it. Cover the liquid with a tight fitting lid so the steam does not escape. Let stand for 20 minutes, then strain. Take 1-3 Tbsp as necessary.

EARACHES/EAR INFECTION
Warm garlic oil due to its antibiotic effect, is excellent for an ear infection. Place 1-2 drops in the ear daily. If both ears are infected, do not use the same dropper for each ear as this may spread the infection. Mullein oil has an anti-inflammatory property and is splendid for the pain. Place 1-2 drops in the ear daily. These two oils together work wonders.

ENEMA – ONION OR GARLIC
This is especially good to fight infection anywhere in the body. It will pull mucus from the colon, kill parasites, aids in hypertension and is a general cleanser of the colon. Blend up garlic (5 or 6 bulbs or equivalent of onion) in 1 cup water. Strain. Add enough water to this solution to equal 2 quarts. For a baby, use 1 small bud to 1 pint of water. Use twice a day for best results.

FOOT BATH
Blend six cloves of garlic in a pint of hot water and let it sit for an hour. Put the feet in a small tub large enough to cover the feet up to the ankles, in water as hot as you can stand it. Add the blended garlic cloves and water. Add more hot water as necessary to keep the bath hot. Soak the feet for 15 minutes. This will treat fungal infections and also the entire system, much like a foot poultice. This is an excellent tonic treatment for fatigue. (This idea is from *The Healing Power of Garlic*).

FUNGAL SKIN INFECTION
Take 3 garlic bulbs, 2 cups of cabbage, 4 onions and 1 potato and crush or finely mince the fresh vegetables. Apply to the skin to fight against infection and will aid in healing. To protect the skin, apply a light coating of vegetable or olive oil before you place these vegetables on the skin. Leave on overnight as a poultice.

GARLIC SYRUP

A recipe for garlic syrup comes from *The Healing Power of Garlic*: "Chop or slice several bulbs of garlic and place it in a clean glass jar. Cover with local, raw, unheated hone. Within a day, the juice from the garlic will mix with the honey. Take the resulting runny syrup for coughs, sore throat, or congestion in the lungs.

HEMORRHOIDS, VAGINAL INFECTIONS, ETC.

"Blend or finely chop a bulb of garlic and pour a quart of boiling water over it. Let it stand for several hours until it is at room temperature. Find a tub just big enough to sit in. Fill it with enough hot water to cover you up to the hips. Add the quart of garlic water along with the blended garlic. Sit in it for ten minutes." *The Healing Power of Garlic*

HIGH BLOOD PRESSURE

Take one teaspoon of blended garlic 5 times daily.

IMMUNE SYSTEM-STRENGTHENS

Garlic is high in selenium which stimulates the immune system, thus being of value in all infections.

LUNGS – STRENGTHENS

Slice onions and garlic, place in honey and soak overnight. Take 1-2 Tablespoons morning and night to strengthen lungs.

MOSQUITOS

Crush raw garlic and stir it into a quart of water. Sprinkle this water over open pools of water with contain mosquito larvae. The garlic mixture will kill them.

MUMPS

Take 2 parts garlic and 1 part onion, chop or grate and mix in hot flax seed tea and charcoal powder. Mix until a thick paste forms and apply hot to a swollen neck or glands.

Grate or chop fresh onion or garlic and mix in a hot tea and drink. Add the chopped or grated onion to warm vegetable oil and apply to a swollen neck.

NASAL CONGESTION
Garlic tea, made by boiling four cups of water, removing from the heat and adding crushed garlic cloves, is reported to relieve nasal stuffiness.

PNEUMONIA
Two garlic bulbs and 3 onion bulbs blended up, and ½ tsp ginger, ½ tsp cayenne pepper, 3 small radish bulbs, and 1/3 tsp of peppermint oil. Add 2 cups of honey and ½ cup fructose. Take ½ tsp as needed.

RINGWORM
Rub fresh garlic juice or garlic oil on the area infected with the ringworm *(Compiler's note: Athlete's Food is a type of Ringworm)*.

SINUSITIS
Grate 2 garlic bulbs and 2 onions. Add ½ tsp peppermint oil, one cup of honey, juice of 2 lemons, 4 Tbsp of horseradish and ½ tsp cayenne pepper. Take ½ tsp as needed.

Combine grated or chopped onion, garlic, horseradish, a little peppermint oil and apple cider vinegar. Apply on cloth over sinuses three times per day.

SPLINTER – REMOVE
Do not attempt to remove splinter from the eyes.
Place garlic paste on a cloth and apply to area with splinter for 5-6 hours. This will loosed the tissue with blisters to open up the blisters to let the splinter out. ***Do not use this if a diabetic.***

STREP THROAT

Chop, dice or grate garlic and onions and use them to make a tea. Gargle with this 2-3 times daily. Drink 1 tsp 4-5 times daily in addition to gargling with the tea.

Also may take one cup of hot water and blend with one clove of garlic. Gargle with this solution every hour until better.

SUNBURN

"Blend three garlic cloves in a quart of cold water. Dip a cloth in this and put on the affected are. Let it stay in place until the heat of the body warms it up, usually about fifteen minutes. Repeat if desired." *The Healing Power of Garlic*

WART – REMOVE

Slice fresh garlic and secure it with a bandage over the wart.

WHOOPING COUGH

2 cups of honey, 1 cup of fructose, 2 Tbsp of olive oil, 1 tsp of cayenne, ½ tsp ginger, 1/3 tsp clove powder, blend up 3 radishes, 2 bulbs of garlic and 2 bulbs of onions. Add juice of 4 lemons. Take 1 tsp as needed.

An old Siberian Remedy for whooping cough is as follows: Chop 5 garlic bulbs and place in 1 quart of soy milk. Boil for 5 minutes and strain. Sweeten with honey to taste. Take 3 oz as needed.

YEAST INFECTIONS – GARLIC SUPPOSITORIES FOR

Quick to make, easy to apply, and very effective, garlic suppositories are a favorite remedy of many women. Carefully peel a clove of garlic and wrap a piece of thick gauze around the garlic. Fold the gauze in half and twist into a tail. It will look like a homemade tampon. Insert the suppository well inside the vaginal cavity. A fresh suppository should be inserted every 3-5 hours. Repeat for 3 days.

RECIPE FOR GARLIC OIL

Peel fresh garlic (4-8 oz.), mince, and put into a wide-mouth glass jar. Add cold-pressed olive oil until the cloves are covered. Close and sit for 3-7 days. Shake it daily. Strain. Put in a dark bottle to store in a cool place. For fevers, intestinal infections, mucus in the stomach, colds and flu, take one teaspoon every hour in a little lemon juice or water. Rub on skin for skin problems.

An alternative preparation would be to let the solution set in the sun for 4-8 hours. Do this when the garlic oil is needed in a hurry.

DOSAGE OF GARLIC

- Capsules – 2 or 3 taken 3 times per day
- Raw cloves – 1-3 at each meal OR 1 a day may be sufficient

HOW TO JUICE

If one has a juicer, the onion may be juiced in it. If garlic is put through, the juicer cannot be washed off and will flavor anything juiced at a later time. When a juicer is not available, place an onion (medium to large) in a blender with approximately ¼ cup of water and blend until juice. Strain and use as directed in the instructions. This may be done with garlic as well.

BIBLIOGRAPHY

Special Thanks
A very special thank you to Mamon Wilson for sharing his knowledge of ways to use onions and garlic in natural remedies.

Balch, James F., M.D., and Phyllis A. Balch, N.C., *Prescription & Dietary Wellness* and *Prescription for Nutritional Healing*

Bergner, Paul, *The Healing Power of Garlic,* Copyright 1996 by Paul Bergner, Prima Publishing, Rocklin, CA. Buy or order at better bookstores or call 1-800-632-8676

Gladstar, Rosemary, *Herbal Healing for Women*

Mayfield, Ann, *Kitchen Apothecary*

McIntyre, Ann, *The Complete Woman's Herbal*

Santilla, Humbart, B.S., N.H., *Natral Healing With Herbs*

Tenny, Louise, M.H., *Today's Healthy Eating and The Health Handbook*

The Natural Medicine Collective, with Rebecca Papas, *The Natural Way of Healing Women's Health.*

Thrash, Agatha, M.D., and Calvin Thrash, M.D., *Home Remedies, Hydrotherapy, Massage, Charcoal and Other Simple Treatments and Natural Healthcare For Your Child.*

Charcoal – The World's Best Adsorbent

What is Charcoal?
Charcoal is the residue left after wood or certain other substances have been burnt. When the wood burns, the gases, resins, proteins and fats, etc. are burnt out leaving the remaining charcoal full of minute holes and crevices which make it brittle and porous. Put simply, Charcoal is charred wood.

What is Adsorption?
Adsorption is attaching onto, rather than absorption, or taking into. Eighty litres of ammonia gas molecules can pack into the crevices of one litre of pulverised charcoal. The molecules are attached to the porous surface of the charcoal. Charcoal is therefore more correctly described as an adsorbent rather than an absorbent.

Activated Charcoal
The ability to activate charcoal did not come until after the turn of the 20th century, but was being used and was recognised as a useful healing agent even its regular state.

Activated charcoal is produced from the controlled burning of wood or bone that is subjected to the action of an oxidising gas such as steam or air at elevated temperatures. Regular charcoal still contains residues from the other elements that were burnt out of it. The process of activating charcoal enhances the adsorptive power by removing the residue and developing an extensive network of fine pores.

When charcoal is activated, the surface area of one cubic centimeter is 1000 square meters! This expanded surface is due to thousands of crevices, pits, grooves, and holes which, when opened out and cleared of residue, make quite a large surface area, hence also expanding the ability to adsorb poisons.

It's Use

Since charcoal is non-toxic and can effectively adsorb a wide variety of poisons, it is of great use as a medicine both internally and externally. If fact, charcoal adsorbs well at body temperature, even better than at high temperatures.

Charcoal has been used as a folk remedy as far back as recorded history. North American Indians used charcoal for the treatment of gas pains long before Europeans settled in the country.

The light and fluffy black powder of charcoal has been used as an officially recognised antidote since the 19th century. Pharmacist P. F. Touery, in 1831, demonstrated the effectiveness of charcoal before the French Academy of Medicine. He swallowed 15 grams of strychnine (ten times the lethal dose) and an equal amount of charcoal (about three tablespoons full) and survived.

Charcoal adsorbs poison when mixed directly with it in the stomach. It would seem unlikely that it could extract poisons after they had entered the gastrointestinal tract or into blood stream. However, recent experiments have shown conclusively that activated charcoal not only adsorbs in the stomach, small intestine and colon, but can attract and draw from the blood back into the gastrointestinal tract where it adsorbs the poisons and inactivates them.

Buying Charcoal

Charcoal is commonly available in tablet or capsule form from health food outlets. Charcoal powder is less readily available perhaps due to it being a bit messier to handle than the tablets.

Commercial tablets are not as concentrated as charcoal capsules or charcoal powder, being about half as effective. In one study, humans took pulverised charcoal powder and prevented absorption of a drug by 73%. Those taking charcoal tablets were able to prevent absorption by only 48%, or roughly half.

Tablets are made from regular charcoal and about one-quarter of the tablet is starch material and other substances used to hold the tablets together. Chewing tablets well before swallowing is essential to increase their effectiveness.

The capsules contain pulverised charcoal, which is usually activated. The activated capsules are roughly twice as potent as the tablets. Briquettes and BBQ charcoals are generally not safe for either external or internal use, as various fillers and chemicals are applied to hold them together and they usually have accelerants for igniting and continues bright burning.

Another point to note is that charred toast and other scorched foods in the kitchen are not healthful – that are not charcoal. These represent charred protein, fats, carbohydrates and mineral salts, the very parts burned away in charcoal, leaving only charred cellulose.

Make your Own
Charcoal can be easily made at home with some basic ingredients and a bit of time. Put pieces of wood in a fireplace or grill them to char the wood well. Even better, if space permits, is burning in a hollow outdoors. After the wood is burning brightly, it should be covered with a large piece of tin with dirt piled over it, forming a dome to exclude air. As the heat continues to burn the wood with decreased oxygen, the soft parts of the wood are burned out first and the hard parts remain, making a good grade of charcoal.

Cut portions from the wood with a sharp knife, or machete. Place these portions into a cloth bag and pound them into coarse granules, then finally into a blender and grind to a fine powder. Remember that this charcoal is not activated and the dosage will need to be about three to four times that of activated charcoal dosages.

Charcoal can be made from a variety of organic materials such as wood pulp, petroleum coke, coals, peat, sawdust, wood char, paper mill waste, bone, and coconut shells. Any kind of wood, such a spine, willow, oak eucalyptus and others, are adequate sources of wood charcoal.

Charcoal made from vegetable materials such as wood and coal contains about 90% carbon whereas bone charcoal contains about 11% carbon, 9% calcium carbonate, and 78% calcium phosphate.

Charcoal maintains its potency for an indefinite period if kept in a closed container. It can even be re-used once or twice by sashing, setline, pouring off the fluid, and drying in the oven at a high temperature (175*C/350*F).

Using Charcoal

Every home should have charcoal on hand as a ready antidote for poisoning, as a cleansing agent in infections, as a room deodorizer, and as a treatment for diarrhea, nausea and vomiting, and many intestinal infections. Skin ulcers, orthopedic casts, bad breath are also helped with use of charcoal. Cleaning the teeth regularly using charcoal instead of toothpaste every so often gets teeth sparkling white, strange and all that it may seem.

It can be safely administered in the home and used by non-professionals. It is harmless if taken into the system accidentally, even in large quantities and there are no ill effects when it comes in contact with the skin.

If poisoning or infection is suspected and the immediate reaction is to use charcoal, there would be no damage done to the body. Even if it did no good, it will not do any harm. Activated charcoal is very well tolerated, even in amounts up to 100 grams (about 1 ¾ cups of pulverized dry powder).

There appears to be no problems with long-term use of charcoal, but as with all treatments it would be recommended that it be used only as needed for acute conditions. The only recommendation for long term use would be if a long-term problem exists, such as gas and odours in colostomy and ileostomy patients.

Some will take a small dosage of charcoal on a regular basis as a problem-preventer. If at all possible though, it would be far better to eliminate any harmful agent entering the body to avoid constant charcoal intake. There are several reasons for this:
1. A dependency usually develops on a remedy rather than an effective remedy being available when trouble strikes.
2. There is a small possibility of interfering with nutrient balance.
3. It does incur some cost and this could be well put to better use.

Internal Use
The oral usage is one tablespoon of powder stirred into a small amount of water. Four capsules of activated charcoal represent about one tablespoon, or eight tablets, or regular charcoal. It is best not taken at mealtimes as food tends to interfere with the best adsorption rate of the charcoal. It has been found that there is approximately a 50% reduction in the effect when the stomach is full.

If a poison is swallowed while food is in the stomach, to be on the safe side, it is recommended to take a volume of charcoal approximately eight to ten times to the estimated weight of the poison swallowed. For best results, use finely powdered charcoal as it can get to the surface of the toxins better than a coarse product.

If there needs to be repetitive doses during the day, a suggested schedule would be to take the first dose upon rising in the morning, another midway between breakfast and lunch, another midway between lunch and tea and at bedtime.

Babies and children accept slurries made of water and powdered activated charcoal quite well. If any problems arise, serve in a fruit juice container, or some opaque container that they cannot see the contents and offer for them to drink with a straw. The fine powder will be easier for a child to get down than chunky grit. Even for adults, it is much easier to swallow in a fine powder form.

External Use

Charcoal is as effective in **drawing poisons and toxins** externally as it is internally. A charcoal compress for a large area such as the abdomen or a knee joint can be made as follows. Mix three tablespoons of cornstarch or ground linseed with one to three tablespoons of charcoal. Stir into one cup of water, set aside for 10-20 minutes to thicken, a little heat will make thickening quicker.

Spread the mixture on to a paper towel of the appropriate size to cover the infected area, about 5 mm thick. Cover this mixture with another paper towel and then apply to the area needing treatment. A square of plastic must then be placed over the compress, with at least 25mm overlap. Cover the entire compress with an old towel to catch any possible leakage, and it also holds it in place. A roller bandage may also be used to hold it in place, pinning or taping to secure properly. This will allow the patient to move about easier.

To make a compress for a **bee sting, spider bite** or other **venomous bite**, mix a spoonful or more of charcoal powder or crush several tablets in plain water (enough to make sufficient paste to cover the area to be treated). Spread the paste on the folded piece of paper toweling large enough to cover the area to be treated and mould the compress to the area. The toweling should be thoroughly moistened with the paste. Cover the compress with a piece of plastic cut from a bread bag, or something of the sort, large enough to cover the compress, plus overlap about 25mm. Secure into place with a snug-fitting garment or bandage.

Be careful in applying a charcoal compress to freshly broken skin. A tattooing effect is possible as the wound heals. There is usually very little need to use a compress of any kind on a fresh open wound as charcoal is used mainly for infection, inflammation and swelling.

The information in this section is drawn from the book *Rx: Charcoal* by Dr. Agatha Thrash, M.D. and Dr. Calvin Thrash, M.D. For detailing of charcoal and treatment plans, we recommend the purchase of this comprehensive books to optimize the use of the world's best and most powerful adsorbent.